**The
Institute
For
Psychoanalysis**

*180 N. MICHIGAN AVENUE
CHICAGO, ILLINOIS 60601*

TERMINAL CARE
Friendship Contracts with
Dying Cancer Patients

Terminal Care

Friendship Contracts with Dying Cancer Patients

by

LOMA FEIGENBERG, M.D.

Associate Professor of Psychiatry (Thanatology)
Radiumhemmet,
Karolinska Hospital,
Stockholm, Sweden

Translated by Patrick Hort, Stockholm

BRUNNER/MAZEL, *Publishers* ● New York

Library of Congress Cataloging in Publication Data

Feigenberg, Loma, 1918-
  Terminal care.

  Translation of Terminalvård.
  A revision of the author's thesis, Karolinska institutet.
  Bibliography: p.
  Includes index.
  1. Terminal care.   2. Death—Psychological aspects.   3.   Psychother-
apy.   4. Cancer—Psychological aspects.   I. Title   [DNLM: 1.
Terminal care—Psychology.   2. Neoplasms—Psychology.   3. Death.
WB310.F297t]
R726.8.F4513   1980   616'.029   79-25904
ISBN   0-87630-224-X

Copyright © 1980 by Loma Feigenberg

Published by
BRUNNER/MAZEL, INC.
19 Union Square
New York, New York 10003

FOR *KAJSA*

Contents

APPENDICES

Foreword

It is especially heartening in these days when any affirmative or original thought must breach the tide of a waning ethos of rebellion, disillusion and mediocrity to find a voice that speaks sensibly and unafraid about death and dying. Given the fact that life is complicated, it follows that dying—a mysterious matrix of living behaviors—is also complex and not reducible to any simplistic set of mini-epochs to be counted on the fingers of one hand. Loma Feigenberg's *Terminal Care* is a book that reflects the extraordinary background of this extraordinary man—oncologist and psychiatrist at Stockholm's famed Karolinska Hospital—and outlines and expands upon the moral, cultural, interpersonal and psychological facets of various dying scenarios. And more than that, it advances fresh ideas in detailing the special features of Dr. Feigenberg's own special way of interacting with persons who are terminally ill.

The subtitle of *Terminal Care* tells us much of its content and thrust: Friendship Contracts with Dying Cancer Patients. In a sense—perhaps growing unconsciously out of Dr. Feigenberg's own charismatic personality—*Terminal Care* rests on an expansion of the psychoanalytic concept of transference, written in large bold type. In his way of doing things, the therapist is the patient's staunch friend and—after carefully explaining this arrangement to both the patient and patient's family members—the therapist devotes himself exclusively to the patient.

Dr. Feigenberg's concise description of his method is clarified, I believe, by a few small emendations, indicated in brackets:

> In order to focus on the psychological needs of the dying person, I deliberately confine myself to the patient and exclude [myself from] all forms of contact with relatives and the regular nursing staff [after carefully explaining to them what the method is].

I am singularly advantaged in writing this Foreword: I have spent several weeks with Dr. Feigenberg in the very Radiumhemmet which he describes in his book, meeting with him every day (yes, Saturdays and Sundays too). He did me the great favor and courtesy of permitting me to sit in with him with several of his patients, both in his consultation room and in their hospital rooms, and I saw for myself how he works.

In candor, when I first read *Terminal Care* (before my salubrious visit), I puzzled over what appeared to me to be perhaps an unnecessarily strong stance about not interacting with the patient's relatives. In actual practice, I can say for myself that Dr. Feigenberg, in a most tender way, encourages their visiting their sick relatives and that, in sum, what he is attempting to do is to focus on the patient, to keep the patient's confidences, to "belong" to the patient, to give the patient a sense of exclusivity and safety (and comfort) with the therapist, and not to "leak" information to the relatives or to get in the middle between them and the patient. Dr. Feigenberg's method may, at first reading, appear somewhat iconoclastic but, in actual practice, it is not at all heretical. It makes eminently good therapeutic sense.

Equally interesting are Dr. Feigenberg's notions about what is special about clinical thanatology, that is, what distinguishes it from ordinary (not-with-dying-patients) psychotherapy. These special features are implied throughout the book. They include the unique nature of the existential confrontation between a therapist and a dying patient, the changes in the dimension of time, the possibility of intense transference, the importance of empathy and flexibility and the special ambience of the dying scene. All these items raise the single question of whether or not clinical thanatology ought to be considered a separate art or discipline from ordinary psychotherapy with non-dying persons. Loma Feigenberg thinks so. And so do I. And so probably will most readers after they have read this singularly important humane and health-giving book. *Terminal Care* is a book of innovative explications, illuminating case histories and fascinating ruminations about the dying process. It is a book which I recommend with enthusiasm and endorse with fervor. Every person who works with dying patients ought to read it.

Edwin S. Shneidman
Professor of Thanatology
University of California at Los Angeles

Preface

This book is written late in the author's professional life. The fact that it is a revision of a book written as an academic thesis may seem still more odd.

My development has been an unusual one, in that I became an oncologist first, then a psychiatrist in order to work in this second capacity in Sweden's major Oncological Department, Radiumhemmet. Although dealing with death and dying was and is only part of my duty, what now is called thanatology has engrossed me for the last ten years.

A need to express my views and experience and even to make thanatology recognized as a professional field in my country made me write the thesis that constitutes the basis of the present work.

Now that this book is published in English, I want to thank the following friends on both sides of the Atlantic who generously helped me in different ways: Johan Cullberg, Marilyn Dunn, Ruth Ettlinger, Robert Fulton, Robert Kastenbaum, and Edwin S. Shneidman. I want to acknowledge the support of the Swedish Cancer Society and to express my admiration of Patrick Hort's translation.

The responsibility for the views expressed is, however, mine only.

And finally—without my wife Kajsa there would have been no book.

LOMA FEIGENBERG

Stockholm
January, 1980

xiii

Introduction

During recent years the problem of death has been brought forward and discussed to an increasing extent in a large part of the world. Many factors, not fully explored, have contributed to this. The subject tends to generate anxiety and perplexity among people in general and especially among professionals. There is a growing demand for proper care of dying persons, the topic of terminal care is being increasingly debated, and various ways for care of the dying have been proposed.

This book describes one particular approach to care of the dying, which I have developed in my work with cancer patients. In order to concentrate on the psychological needs of the dying person, I deliberately focus my energies: Except for typically only one orientation session with the close relatives of the patient, in which the nature of my relationship or "contract" with the patient is made clear, I limit my contacts to the patient alone. In this way I attempt to become his* personal, special, confidential doctor around the topics or problems relating to his being terminally ill (or anything else that the patient wishes to discuss). Thus, the relationship between me and the patient is intensified and a friendship contract is established.

---

* A comment about my use of the pronoun "he" is needed. Although I recognize the inequity of using the male pronoun for the therapist or patient, I have done so for convenience and readability.

The term "friendship contract" is admittedly debatable.
We usually do not make contracts about friendship. It is the
need for complete seclusion with a dying human being in this
setting which makes a contract necessary. In this friendship
the emotional side is emphasized. Unlike most friendships,
which tend to develop slowly and last for years, this relationship, for the very reason that the patient is dying, is established easily and quickly and will have a limited duration.

To describe this particular psychological care of dying, the
word *method* will often be used in this book, for the sake of
brevity. What I have in mind, however, is, rather, an approach or the implementation of an ideology of care. In order to present this ideology and make it alive to the reader,
I will describe my approach to care of dying cancer patients
from various viewpoints and on different levels and analyze
the effect of my approach on all concerned.

Each part of the book—theoretical comments upon clinical thanatology (what I call dimensions), five case histories
about dying patients I have treated, a detailed description of
the ongoing contact with dying patients, discussions of the
therapist's qualifications, the assessment and application of the
method in medical care—all express, in different ways, my
views on psychological care of the dying.

THE AIM OF THE BOOK

The aim of this book can be expressed more systematically
in the following points:

> *To present a special method for psychological termi-
> nal care.* Different people—clinical thanatologists—
> have developed methods for care of the dying along dif-
> ferent lines and often without exact specifications. Here
> one, admittedly a special one, will be described in de-
> tail. It is wholly concentrated on psychological care and
> on the terminal phase of life.

To reveal effects of the method. Effects of the method can hardly be verified scientifically. Instead, my aim has been to describe what happens and thereby present the influence of this approach on those concerned. The phenomenon of death inevitably engages everyone emotionally. In order to evaluate effects of this method one must, therefore, do what one can to catch and record the impressions not only of the dying patient but also of relatives, staff and the therapist himself. The exclusion of the patient's family is evidently a somewhat problematic measure. Besides presenting the rationale of doing so, this approach will, however, indirectly give a picture of the difficulties and strains in general for those nearest the dying. An exhaustive description of such a total effect is not feasible, but my account of the method will include an attempt to suggest, establish and evaluate the experience of all the persons concerned. It may even be worth discussing the reactions of the readers of this book.

To contribute to knowledge of the psychology of dying. Close psychological contact with dying people throws the reactions of the individual, the course and psychodynamics of dying, and the dying person's experience of approaching death into very clear relief. Using my experience with the patients described here, I shall attempt to illuminate the psychological side of death and dying.

To illustrate and influence the role of medical personnel in care of the dying. Although the method presented here is special in several respects, much of what is depicted in attitudes and behavior towards the patients, as well as in the method's effects on those involved, applies to other terminal situations, too. Experience of this method should also be applicable in other forms of terminal care and be useful to professionals of various orientations, doctors, nurses, social workers and others.

To contribute to social and psychodynamic psychiatry. Traditional psychiatry deals in the main with research into and the care of certain psychiatric disturbances and groups of diseases that have been brought together for historical and other reasons. It almost entirely ignores people's difficulties in accepting life on its own terms and their reactions to loneliness, poverty, illness and death. Psychiatry at present seldom becomes involved in the mental suffering of people faced with a severe disease or the threat of death. It is, therefore, unacquainted with much of the pain and suffering in the human condition and, accordingly, lacks insight into a wide field of knowledge and experience. Psychiatrists and psychologists with a social and dynamic orientation are, however, paying increasing attention to such questions. This work is intended to be a contribution to social and psychodynamic psychology.

To illustrate death as an existential problem. We all have a highly composite emotional and cognitive relation to death as a phenomenon. Death has fundamental effects on life in general, as well as on the life of each individual. Death can be seen in a global, an international and even a political context. Our conception of death influences social structures, pervades political attitudes and colors the psychology of the individual. In a sense, death, like life, is constantly with us.

Even when describing a particular approach, used on a limited number of patients in a specific medical institution, one is continuously confronted with the elusive and complex nature of death. In a number of contexts I shall, therefore, return, partly indirectly, to matters which are associated with the universal question: "What is death?"

To broaden the scope of medical practice. The medical profession is mainly oriented towards prevention or cure of diseases. The fact that sooner or later cure is impossible to achieve and that everybody will have to face death after a shorter or longer period of dying is denied or evaded. The opposite stand is at the core of my ideology. Through this work I want to contribute to an integration of psychological and medical care of the dying into medical care in general.

MY PROFESSIONAL BACKGROUND

My *training* as a physician is twofold. As an oncologist I soon became interested in the psychological problems in the care of cancer patients. As this line of work was then in its infancy and hardly existed in Sweden, it seemed worthwhile obtaining extensive training in radiotherapy and a corresponding insight into psychiatry. After seven or eight years as an oncologist at Radiumhemmet (the major cancer unit in Stockholm) at the Karolinska Hospital, I worked for about as long at the Department of Psychiatry at the same hospital.

My psychiatric training has been relatively conventional and eclectic but I have tried to give it a psychodynamic turn by means of study trips, wide reading and supervision when necessary from an experienced psychoanalyst. I do not have a personal psychoanalytic training.

For several years my work brought me into contact with the psychiatric clientele in the metropolitan area of Stockholm. I have acquired experience of psychopharmacological and electroconvulsive treatments and grappled with problems in the field of social psychiatry, besides undertaking psychotherapies of varying duration, some of them under supervision.

It is worth noting that during my early years at the Department of Psychiatry I hardly met a single patient whose problem involved a reaction to somatic disease. At that time, the early '60s, the doctors at Radiumhemmet, for instance, saw little reason to refer patients to the Department of Psychiatry on account of psychic reactions to cancer or reactions associated with the treatment. Faced with a referral of such a problem, the psychiatric doctors were equally hesitant and uncertain.

From the mid-'60s onwards, at the Department of Psychiatry, particularly its outpatient department, I gradually devoted myself more and more to cancer patients, who were referred to me by doctors at Radiumhemmet.

Since 1972 I have been what in the United States corresponds to Associate Professor of Psychiatry stationed at Radiumhemmet with the task of handling the psychological care of cancer patients. I am thus on the staff of the Department of Psychiatry and can take part in its lectures, symposia and organizational meetings. I am also entitled in principle to admit patients to this department.

At an organizational level my work became incorporated with the other aspects of clinical oncology at Radiumhemmet and designated the Psychosomatic Department. Besides my hospital duties, I have a teaching commitment in psychiatry and oncology for medical students.

The problem of death and thanatological work captured my interest as I got to know more and more cancer patients and at the same time became more closely acquainted with my oncological colleagues. I started to observe and analyze my own as well as their reactions to dying patients and to death. A varying amount of my time is now devoted to care of the dying.

Over the years I have had opportunities to lecture and hold seminars on the problem of death and dying with various categories of hospital staff in Sweden. I have conducted courses in terminal care at the Karolinska Hospital, ranging from brief introductions, e.g., for intensive-care personnel, to extensive one-year courses with practical and theoretical training for different categories of medical staff.

I have, accordingly, acquired a special interest in thanatology as a result of reading about the subject, encountering dying patients and also observing the attitudes of doctors and the hospital organization to dying and death (Feigenberg, 1971a, b, c, 1974; Feigenberg & Fulton, 1976a, b, 1977).

My *workplace* (office, consulting room, etc.) in Radiumhemmet is a few minutes' walk from the Department of

Psychiatry. Consequently, I am in an excellent position to meet and talk when necessary with the staff of both departments. It is easy for patients, as well as doctors, at Radiumhemmet to find their way to the Psychosomatic Department, which the patients regard as an integrated part of Radiumhemmet. I always let patients know that I am a psychiatrist, but because of my address and the location of my reception office I am regarded as one of the doctors at Radiumhemmet.

Radiumhemmet is organized into two departments, one general and the other gynecologic, with 91 and 44 beds, respectively. The outpatient side has expanded and is now very large; about 60,000 patients a year are seen in the two departments combined. In addition, some 50,000 visits are made for radiation or chemotherapy.

The Psychosomatic Department has the task of taking care of cancer patients with psychological-psychiatric problems that are related to their disease, treatment, rehabilitation and so on. The patients are referred by doctors at Radiumhemmet. The reasons for referral are usually a psychological or psychosomatic problem, psychiatric symptom, deviant behavior or, for instance, conflicts between patients and personnel.

On various occasions my colleagues at Radiumhemmet and I have discussed forms of cooperation and principles for the treatment of cancer patients with psychological complaints. At conferences we have considered the work of the Psychosomatic Department and agreed about routines, e.g., for the referral of patients. I consider it particularly important that the patient be informed that the referral is for a psychiatric consultation. If the patient is in the least doubtful or hesitant about this, I expect the referring doctor to explain that an appointment with a psychiatrist does not mean that the patient is considered to be mentally ill or has behaved unsuitably in any way. The following points should be made clear to the patient.

Unrest, anxiety, grief or distress on account of serious illness, depression in the face of major surgery and difficulties in adjusting to hospital care are common and understandable reactions. Hospital staff tend to have too little time for the patients and perhaps lack of training in the proper psychological handling of these problems. It is for this reason that the patient is being referred to a doctor at Radiumhemmet who is a specialist in psychiatry as well as in cancer. On occasion a patient will reject a proposed referral to a psychiatrist and this naturally has to be respected.

My position and status as psychiatrist at Radiumhemmet are equal to the somatic doctors and give me full right of decision about patient care. Having received a referral, I decide how the contact is to be arranged, the duration of treatment and so on. I am free to prescribe medicine and arrange for examinations at Radiumhemmet and I naturally have access to all case records. In other words, my work is integrated with the institution's routines and is based on open, mutual cooperation with my colleagues on the somatic side. A written reply to a referral is drafted as soon as the situation has been properly assessed. I usually manage to have a short, personal talk with the referring doctor in order to discuss the situation, agree on a joint plan of action or present my view of the psychological situation. It is also agreed that I, in turn, shall be kept informed about the course of the disease and about major steps or changes in the plan of treatment. Besides the referred cases, I can take on patients at my own discretion whom I meet on rounds or who contact me personally.

The medical health service in Sweden is such that inpatients at a hospital do not pay and outpatients pay only a fixed, limited amount to the hospital. This gives me the freedom to decide which patients I take on and how much time I want to devote to them without having to consider their financial situation.

TERMINAL CARE
Friendship Contracts with Dying Cancer Patients

Part I
THE STUDY OF DYING

Chapter 1

Clinical Thanatology

Death has been a central problem since time immemorial in religion, philosophy and ethics, besides recurring continuously as a theme in literature, art and music. The problem of death has featured differently in the cultural pattern of different societies. Some writers refer to cultures that are death-denying, death-opposing, death-desiring or death-accepting (Borkenau, 1955, Pattison, 1974a). Attitudes toward death have been influenced by many complex factors and conflicting forces in different cultures or subcultures. Feelings and attitudes about death, ways of coping with the process of dying, burial rites and rituals, the place of death in everyday life— all these have contributed to the patterns—with their social, psychological, religious and cultural determinants—that have arisen, predominated, died away and been succeeded by others in different periods and different countries (Aries, 1974).

The term "death system" has been proposed by Kastenbaum (1972) as a comprehensive label for the network of thoughts, conceptions, feelings, actions, behaviors, customs and usages that occur in connection with death in a particular culture at a particular time, the aim being to obtain an overall picture that could serve as a starting point for thinking and research about dying and death.

5

As in a large part of the Western world, attitudes toward death in Sweden during the present century can be characterized on the whole as death-denying (Feigenberg & Fulton, 1977), but this situation seems to be changing. Consequently, our present death system is particularly complex and prone to conflicting tendencies, emotions and attitudes. There are groups who display a mystical, superstitious involvement in questions dealing with death and dying, manifested, for instance, in criticism of the medical service's professional work with dying persons.

Death is now, in this confusing situation, the subject of a newly-aroused scientific interest. A discipline is being built up which people regard as new, although death has in fact engaged man throughout the ages.

THANATOLOGY

The scientific study of everything that has to do with death is beginning to be known as thanatology (from Thanatos, the god of death in Greek mythology). Thanatology has been defined in different ways (Weisman, 1972, 1974). One may ask whether the aspects of something so many-faceted as death should, in fact, be given a comprehensive name. After all, the problem of death is far from being a coherent, well-defined subject. One of the reasons for promoting the term thanatology has been to give the subject status on a par with other disciplines. Perhaps there has also been a desire—albeit a debatable one—to de-dramatize the emotional side of death and dying or to de-romanticize (Shneidman, 1971) death. The term thanatology can also be interpreted as an attempt to place a scientific screen around the reality of death. It seems reasonable to suppose that the term thanatology will change its content as time passes, becoming more exact, restricted or extended. In this book I shall use it as a label for the "new" conscious effort to investigate, systematize and apply knowledge from various fields to death, dying and related phenomena. Contemporary thanatology is a young discipline. It reflects a swing from a period of denying death and is dominated by modern sociological, psychological and philosophical (e.g., existentialist) theories and knowledge, as they are applied to the problem of death. It is hardly surprising that the publications in which thanatology is discussed and quoted mainly have appeared during or since the first world war. Their background comprises the two world wars, the social and cultural climate of the inter-war period and post-war development. During this time our death system has been influenced by many complex factors. The millions of lives lost in these wars, the mass extermination of populations on a previously unknown scale, the gap between rich and poor countries, the threat of nuclear war and global pollution of the environment, as well as tremendous social progress, greatly increased life expectancy and major medical discoveries—all these have helped to shape the Western view of death and left their mark on thanatology today.

CLINICAL THANATOLOGY

Thanatology is a multidisciplinary science. One cannot separate its psychological, medical, social, cultural, anthropological and other components for the simple reason that death, like life, is "multi-disciplinary."

Clinical thanatology is emerging (Shneidman, 1973) as a special field, applying thanatological insights in practical clinical work. Clinical thanatology is chiefly concerned with three matters: 1) care of the dying, 2) suicide and its prevention, and 3) grief and care of the bereaved.

TERMINAL CARE

Care of the dying is now being discussed and researched in a purposeful manner by clinical thanatologists. The task of providing care for dying persons is being left more and more to the medical profession, at least in industrial countries. This terminal care, as it is frequently known, should cater not only for the dying person but also for the bereaved and the personnel who look after these groups. When planning terminal care, one must draw on the knowledge and experience to be found in clinical thanatology. At present, when faced with these difficult situations, medical personnel tend to be hesitant and ambivalent (Feigenberg & Fulton, 1977).

The general tardiness about planning specifically for better care of the dying is being countered in some parts of the world by projects with various forms of terminal care. But these still amount to no more than isolated attempts by a research group, an individual researcher or a clinic. The medical profession as a whole has hardly started to consider the general question of the type of care which should be provided for the dying. It is difficult to find any specific standards for the content of terminal care, although a preliminary attempt to define "Standards of Care for the Terminally Ill" was made in 1974 at a meeting of theoretical and clinical thanatologists at Columbia, Maryland (Kastenbaum, 1975b, c, 1976).

It is difficult to establish just where research and development in terminal care stand at present. Terminal care is a part of clinical thanatology, which in turn is only one sector of thanatology. Scientific work connected with thanatology is being undertaken in a wide range of disciplines, with disparate starting points, histories and methods.

The renewed interest in terminal care and the frequently fierce emotional discussions which it arouses are certainly stimulating but they complicate a balanced assessment of what we can do and what we know. There are relatively few weighty scientific works specifically on care of the dying. All over the world people who are dying are receiving terminal care, though its quality varies and it lacks a professional definition. Knowledge is desperately needed, but it can be difficult to find. Modern thanatological literature dates back approximately to the first world war. It has become increasingly prolific and multifarious, particularly since the '50s. In countries like Sweden, where so far there has been little interest in the scientific study of death, it is almost impossible to obtain most of the relevant publications. A survey of thanatological literature is presented in Appendix I.

Various methods of terminal care have been developed by individual researchers or institutions. Their publications have certain shortcomings, partly because clinical thanatology is still in its infancy and partly because of the special nature of all work with death and care of the dying. Those writing about terminal care are liable to be biased by the circumstances of their work. Their experience is limited to the patients available and the results will be conditioned by whether these are persons who have attempted suicide, suffered a heart attack or are dying of cancer. The account will also be influenced by the personality of the clinicians, their attitudes toward religion and toward death. This, of course, is partly inevitable and fully understandable, but it is frequently overlooked by the authors themselves, as well as by the reader.

On top of this there is the circumstance that death, although unique, is in a sense a banal event. There is a tendency to generalize research findings and observations because they happen to be valid in a particular situation. When describing a psychological method for care of the dying it is easy to believe that one's conclusions are applicable to all dying persons on the grounds that all persons die.

The method of presentation and the level of abstraction in works on terminal care may make it difficult for persons engaged in the practical care of dying patients to find clear, exact information and guidance. The student of clinical thanatology is often introduced to specialized philosophical, religious or psychological systems and theories but gets only vague, diffuse instructions regarding practical therapeutic management. The reader wishing to adopt a particular technique or approach usually has to find out for himself what he can apply. There may be very little information about, say, the indications and contraindications that have been employed, what effects a particular measure had on the parties concerned, what qualifications are expected for the clinician, and for which patients a particular method is intended.

Suppose, by way of an illustration, that three prominent clinical thanatologists such as Kübler-Ross, Shneidman and Weisman were to handle one and the same patient or that a person providing terminal care went to these three for advice. Although they have all written extensively about care of the dying, we would still be rather at a loss to tell how each of them would act, their reasons for taking a particular line, how they would proceed in various situations and what would be "best" for the dying person.

In order to promote a discussion and analysis of different methods for terminal care, I have presented in Appendix III a list or scheme of problems or items which should be considered in works about psychological terminal care.

Chapter 2

My Thanatology

This presentation of my fundamental views on death and dying is, in my opinion, one way to illuminate my approach to care of the dying. The review includes comments on and opinions about relevant basic clinical thanatological literature, as well as experience and insights from discussions with clinical thanatologists; however, the main foundation is my own experience during work with dying patients. My thoughts about dying and care of the dying have evolved over the years and are bound to undergo further development and modification as my work with the dying continues. Each new relationship with a dying patient influences me, engages my thoughts and yields new experiences. Meanwhile, I grow older and this also means that, as with anyone else, my views about dying and death change.

I shall concentrate on the subject of this book—dying and care of the dying—almost leaving aside the closely related subject of death, for it is important when discussing terminal care to distinguish between dying—the process leading up to death—and death in the sense of not existing. It need hardly be said, however, that the characteristics of dying are closely bound up with the fact that it ends in death.

In describing my view of the problems of dying, I shall be

11

less concerned with thanatological theory than with practical clinical work with the dying individual. The frame of reference, level of abstraction and degree of generalization one chooses are naturally important here. What I want to express is the whole emotional world of the dying person. The experience of illness, suffering and death is so comprehensive that it will always be difficult to convey in full.

Many of those who have worked with psychological care of the dying and whose contributions are discussed in Appendix I have a fundamental opinion about the psychological significance of dying. Several of them have described this systematically (e.g., Weisman, 1975; Shneidman, 1973; Pattison, 1974a).

My starting point for this presentation of my views is the special approach which I have adopted for care of the dying. My ideology of care is, however, as far as I can see applicable and relevant in terminal care in general.

I first consider 1) dying as a phase of life and look at it in relation to past and future time; then against this background I suggest 2) dimensions for systematizing work with the dying.

DYING AS A PHASE OF LIFE

During life there is always a present, a past and a future. Accordingly, existence for a dying person consists of three periods: 1) what is happening now, namely dying, 2) what has happened, namely life up to now, and 3) what is going to happen, namely death and that which comes after death, however this may be conceived.

Whereas these categories are seldom given more than a passing thought during our lives, the mind of a dying person is dominated by thoughts, feelings and fantasies about death in this altered perspective. Dying can therefore be described in the light of these divisions. One cannot write about any one of them without considering the other two, but for clarity's sake they are discussed separately here. Disregarding chronology, I shall start with dying, as this is our focal point.

Dying

The situation, briefly, is that during a limited period an individual, who has functioned socially, has been active in a network of emotional relationships, has been mobile and in control of himself, with ties in an occupation, family and community, is transformed into what we refer to as dying. It is natural that attempts have been made to systematize and subdivide this phase. The pattern of communication among cancer patients has been studied by Abrams (1966) in relation to the terminal course of the disease. A distinction between a terminal and a preterminal period has been proposed in geriatric studies (Weisman & Kastenbaum, 1968; Isaacs et al., 1971), which is, in my opinion, meaningful for dying in general. Various "dying trajectories" have been described, with a systematic account of their different effects on all concerned (Glaser & Strauss, 1968).

The division into stages which Kübler-Ross (1969) has presented (see p. 138) equates each stage with a particular form of defense against an awareness of approaching death, the final phase being acceptance. This division into stages is now being questioned. From work with dying patients I have the impression that dying is characterized by an unceasing alternation between different forms of behavior and reactions. One encounters a mesh of situations and feelings, with anxiety, depression, revolt or resignation predominating. Consequently, such a comprehensive process as dying can hardly be subdivided solely in terms of defense mechanisms. There is much evidence (Kastenbaum, 1975a) that several other factors leave their mark on the behavior and experiences of dying persons, e.g., the nature of the disease, the patient's ethnic background, the personality, maturity and life-style of the dying person, his age and sex, environment and social situation. It is significant that psychological-psychiatric terminology as well as common speech have few descriptive words for the variety of emotions and modes of reaction to dying. Most of what happens is referred to as anxiety, depression or some such label.

Some writers (e.g., Pattison, 1967) have suggested that death and dying should be regarded as a crisis. It is not always entirely clear whether they mean a developmental or a traumatic crisis. The core of the crisis concept, according to some authors, is that current crisis reminds the individual about the final, overwhelming, unavoidable threat that looms in the background. Others argue that living through a crisis (so that this is resolved and one adapts to the trauma) makes a person more mature and perhaps better equipped to meet the final "crisis" (Cullberg, 1975). The problem has been analyzed thoroughly by Kastenbaum (1975a), who concludes that death is not inevitably a crisis. The process of dying may be a period of crisis for many people but not for everyone.

I must admit that I used to be attracted by the idea of regarding dying as a crisis, partly for purely didactic and pragmatic reasons (Feigenberg, 1971c). There has been a growing interest, in Sweden as elsewhere, in the concept of crisis and in crisis intervention even in the context of medical care. By applying this frame of reference to dying, I saw a possibility of getting the various levels of hospital staff interested in care of the dying. After several years work with the dying, however, I am now very doubtful whether it is meaningful to equate death with the crises that are the usual concern of modern crisis intervention. There is an obvious risk that this will involve an undesirable simplification of the problems of dying.

The concept of crisis, as far as I can see, presupposes that a person is confronted with a real external event. This event exceeds his psychological resources and adaptabilities, creating in him a state of tension and anxiety that activates former problems and conflicts. It is characteristic that the crisis wanes and life continues with the person either more mature (if the solution of the crisis is psychologically appropriate) or wounded to a varying degree. Even in somatic care there is a tendency to regard more and more situations as crises.

Death is experienced as an external event by some dying persons but as an "enemy within" by others. Terminal therapy neither can nor should aim at adaption in the future. There is no future and the problem therefore concerns the patient's ability to live *now,* facing the threat of the inevitable. Consequently, I do not consider crisis to be an adequate designation for dying.

The period's limits. Dying starts at a certain point in time and ends when the person dies. Its duration varies from fractions of a second to hours, days, weeks and occasionally months. A patient may have been ill for years before he starts dying; one can be ill and dying simultaneously. But the period is limited and its end-point is clear; the outcome is given. This limit is a threat to most persons, including those who are balanced and calm about what awaits them after death.

The period's starting point varies with the definition of dying. In the *philosophical* sense it can be said that to some extent we die continuously and thus are dying from the moment of birth. This idea has little relevance in practical care of the sick. *Sociologically* it has been shown (Sudnow, 1967) that in a hospital the doctors make the decision concerning when someone is to be regarded as dying. The scientific foundation for these predictions is very weak and the care provided becomes a not entirely reliable fulfillment of a prophecy.

From the *medical* point of view it has been considered that a person is dying if he has a particular disease or is in a particular phase of a disease that usually leads to death. It is a mistake to mix up disease and death. Death is not a disease and cannot be described solely in medical-biological terms. We are by tradition most familiar with the biological side of dying and death and this is usually our only frame of reference —hence the unwillingness to change our outlook. But dying does also have a *psychological* aspect and at the present stage of life this is wholly dominant. The biological component becomes increasingly uniform, characterized by unspecific symptoms such as fatigue, emaciation and pain, whereas the psychological situation becomes increasingly varied, engaging and full of emotional experiences. When patients have reached a stage where doctors definitely consider they are dying, it is often too late for psychological measures. Most of what we have learned about the psychology of dying derives from studies in the preterminal phase (Weisman, 1977).

In the following account, the term dying refers to the whole psychosocial process, which is, of course, linked to the biological development, though the two by no means always correspond to each other. This is why it is basically the patient himself who is the first to sense or perceive that he is no longer sick but dying. And as the context is psychological, close relatives are often soon aware of the change, too. In the hospital, a good psychological relationship is required to detect when dying starts, so that the patient, instead of suffering the anxiety of keeping his insight to himself, has the confidence to share it with us. Interesting possibilities are afforded by basing the prognosis on psychosocial factors during the course of dying (Worden et al., 1974; Pattison, 1974b; Bruhn et al., 1974; Weisman & Worden, 1975).

To register dying—its beginning and course—one needs understanding of the psychosocial aspects; also, it is the central importance of these psychosocial aspects in dying which explains why psychological measures can be used to assist, accompany and support a dying person.

Changes proceed on every level. For the patient, everything changes during the brief period of dying. In every respect he proceeds from the familiar, the habitual and often secure to something that is unknown, impossible to conceive of and often anxiety-provoking. These changes, moreover, occur continuously, sometimes gradually, calmly but relentlessly, sometimes abruptly and unexpectedly.

Another central aspect of dying, which in itself is full of upheavals, is that changes take place all the time in the dying person's memory, feelings and thoughts about the past and the life he has lived, as well as in his dreams, fears and hopes about the death that lies ahead. And all these shifts, changes and upheavals may take place more or less simultaneously and are interwoven. Most of this happens internally; what we observe and record are reflections.

● *New symptoms* may appear in connection with the disease or its complications. Everyone knows that they are bound to come, no one can do anything to prevent or cure them. Certain unspecific symptoms, such as pain and difficulty in breathing, may completely preoccupy the patient and must be repulsed with every means at our disposal. But others, which may be signs that the underlying disease is progressing, become increasingly insignificant. It is, therefore, irrelevant to try to demonstrate new metastases, or to detect changes on x-rays or in the results of electrocardiograms and laboratory tests.

● *The dying person's view of his earlier life* and his relationships with others changes all the time. Loving ties are broken, horizons close in. This elicits tension, agitation and anxiety, as well as revolt, grief and submission.

● *The attitude toward what lies ahead*—ideas, fantasies and fears about what lies in the hereafter—likewise changes during this period. An earlier faith or hope may suddenly fail, or other feelings may unexpectedly awake and lead to new interpretations of what life is about. Some persons have kept such questions at a distance and may now find reassurance in being able to express and follow a conviction that everything ends with death, that afterwards there is nothing.

● *The manner of dying,* the way in which one meets death and how this will be remembered, means a great deal to many. One cannot be sure how others will remember a person until he has died. Many have painful recollections of how the memory of their parents or relatives was clouded by death-bed scenes. They know that their relatives entertain similar fears.

What Lies in the Past

The individual has been formed all through the period, short or long, that preceded dying. Heredity and environment, emotional and other experiences have all contributed to his development. While a person is dying, everything connected with his earlier life is important because he is in the act of losing it.

● Each person has an *identity* and a *personality,* with all his unique and banal characteristics. One can die at any age. Since we develop in innumerable respects from birth onwards, life must mean different things at the ages of five, 35 and 80. The significance of death and how one feels and thinks about it also evolve, though we know very little about this. In a large number of respects, therefore, dying must involve different burdens, conflicts and questions depending on the individual's maturity, experience and age.

● Physical and spiritual development may have been "normal" or deviant. The patient may have been *healthy or sick* in body and soul. Former problems, illnesses and suffering surface and become significant when a person is dying.

● Everyone has entertained *ideals, dreams and hopes* about what he wants to do with his life. It is the things that have not been achieved which are most painful now. It is important to have an opportunity to talk about them and for some things there may still be time.

● Everyone has *relations* with other people, relations colored by love, indifference or hate, often a mixture of all these. The ties may lie in the same or other generations, as well as with the same or the opposite sex. They may concern persons who are already dead, the patient's own and others' children. These relationships now lose their importance and all these ties have to be broken. This induces anxiety, guilt, grief and despair.

● Most people have belonged to some political, religious or occupational *community* and have had one or several types of *work*. For many this may have been the most meaningful aspect of life.

● A *social identity* is developed during life and this forms the individual, giving a feeling of security and comradeship or, on the contrary, rejection and alienation. One may have settled into a social environment or struggled against it.

● Life for some is full of *setbacks* and struggle. Solitude, poverty and isolation are the lot of many. Large numbers of people have experienced catastrophes, war and concentration camps or been obliged to leave their country or their home environment for political and social reasons. Such matters color the experience of dying and how one accepts or resists death.

The importance of all these and many other factors that have shaped our lives should not be underestimated when a person is dying. Each of these factors contributes to the significance of dying and the whole of its psychosocial form and course; they constitute the important matters that one would now like to share with someone.

What Lies Ahead

Death and what may happen thereafter—the implacable future for a dying person—occupy a large part of the patient's feelings and thoughts.

A common thanatological conundrum is: Which frightens us most—dying or death? Many writers take sides very decidedly. I find such debates incomprehensible. The concepts of dying and death are so elusive and complex that it is hard to see how one can possibly distinguish what people in general, or what the individual, whether healthy or dying, is most alarmed by or fears most. The fact that a person happens to talk more about one than the other does not necessarily mean very much.

Conceptions of *death* find expression in individual fantasies and dreams, such as personifications of death (Kastenbaum & Aisenberg, 1972). During a close personal contact a picture can be formed of what death may mean for the individual. Many people have visions of annihilation, torment and solitude, but one also encounters positive aspects. Death may be longed for, not just because life has been hard but because death may represent a form of completion, be associated with the hope of reunion with the beloved who has gone before, or arouse an emotional (libidinous) expectation. Deep down, the feelings of most people about death are ambivalent.

Few people are entirely neutral in their attitude toward what awaits us *after death*. Consciously or unconsciously, we circle round the subject with dreams and fantasies, hopes and fears. Some organize life after death in accordance with a religious system, while others see it as a "nothingness" where they no longer exist.

Lifton is a contemporary thinker who is deeply familiar with the most alarming realities of our times, having studied people's experiences of war, mass extermination and natural disasters. He substitutes a "need for a symbolic immortality" for Freud's notion of our subconscious immortality (p. 217). According to Lifton (1973), this symbolic immortality consists of five modes: 1) the biological, whereby we live on through our children, 2) the theological, which counts on a physical or spiritual "life" after death, 3) immortality through creativity, manifested in a life's work, 4) immortality with and through nature, and finally 5) experiential transcendence. Most psychological schools ascribe a far-reaching formative significance to birth and experiences in our early years. I find it difficult to believe that the knowledge that we shall die does not have a corresponding influence on our life and our perception. Lifton (1976) is perhaps the first to make a major attempt at creating a psychological system which incorporates death and images of death.

These reflections about life after death obviously touch on questions that are of crucial importance for persons who are dying. Some have thought them over during their lives and may have a firmly rooted opinion. Others are unprepared for and frightened by their emergence. As mentioned earlier, our thoughts and feelings about what happens afterwards presumably undergo a change during the process of dying, creating periods of calm and assurance or agitation and anxiety.

DIMENSIONS OF DYING

Death comes to us all and is, therefore, in a sense banal and commonplace. But as each life is unique, so is its conclusion. In this section I shall describe what takes place on the psychological or human plane and what one aims at when trying to participate in, understand and even share another person's dying. This description should be seen in the light of the altered perspective, outlined above, that life acquires while dying.

I have chosen to formulate a number of dimensions, spectra or polarities which have proved relevant for my work during relationships with persons who are dying. These dimensions, which serve as the basis of questions which I ask myself continuously during such a contact, are provisional. The intention is neither to include every conceivable one, which would be impossible, nor to have distinct boundaries between them. On the contrary, these dimensions are related and fuse more and more as death approaches. With as much empathy and flexibility as possible, one must try to feel one's way in the psychological sphere, understand needs and find means of meeting them. One way of getting through is a dialogue on every level, nonverbal as well as verbal. Another is to use one's fantasy and powers of discernment. Interest in and interpretation of the patient's dreams may prove fruitful. If one strives for closeness and frankness—genuine friendship—the time comes during the process of dying when all these forms of communication or contact amount, in a sense, to the same thing.

Time

Time is in a way the most important dimension, since time and death are linked together. The thought of death presupposes time. We have had a past and look forward to a future, knowing that in this future there will be death.

An irrevocable series of changes, from what has been to what may come, takes place along the dimension we call time. Time is by no means a simple concept. One can distinguish between chronological, biological and subjective (existential) time. When a person is dying, the very passage of time creates anxiety. Moreover, time does not pass uniformly and the experience of sudden accelerations or decelerations creates insecurity and a feeling of helplessness.

The habitual and conventional idea of chronological time as a linear, everlasting process is now broken up by the patient and the medical staff into sections, a relevant measure being the intervals between meals, nursing shifts, visits or pain-killing injections. The perception of chronologcal time alters and disintegrates in the process of dying.

Existential time is the expression of the personal meaning of what happens to a human being in the present. Existential time cannot be measured. It is its quality or significance that can be registered and compared. We are *in* existential time. Future belongs to chronological time. All that is left to the dying person is the situation of being dying and his existential time. This time is filled with convulsive experiences and becomes increasingly disconnected from chronological time, which loses its significance.

In the relationship between past and future time, dying involves major upheavals. More and more of what has been, and to some extent still is, loses its importance, pales and is distorted. The future, always an illusion, is now truly an illusion in quite another sense, at the same time as the horizon closes in and there ceases to be any future at all. Hospital routines are not designed at present to meet the dying patient in this dimension and consider his conception of time. In our own interest we divide up and adhere to chronological time. This may give the staff a sense of security but it accentuates the helplessness of the patient and the discrepancy between chronological and subjective time.

It is important that the therapist get to know the patient's perception of time, when and why it fluctuates or is broken up. He must accept this and try to keep in touch as far as possible, instead of criticizing or letting the patient know that he is "wrong." The dying person is *not* wrong; his perception of time is neither wrong nor right—it simply *is*.

"Inside Here—Out There"

The dying person loses interest in his illness as such. He very seldom mentions its name, the possibilities of treatment or what examinations may have shown. He is engaged in something much more important. He is dying. In one sense the patient's thoughts are bound up with the original disease, in that they may dwell on whether death is somewhere "out there" or "inside." Bacterial infections naturally represent a death that comes from outside. The same applies if one has been wounded by a bullet. Most cancer patients see the threat —the enemy—within them and death is "inside here." Many other diseases, e.g., the cardiovascular ones, feature in fantasies as both "inside here and out there."

The worse a person becomes, the more prone he will be to locate death internally. When subconscious ideas, dreams and fantasies come to light in a close relationship with a patient, it can be very valuable to understand even the spatial dynamics that dying persons associate with death.

Denial and Acceptance

It is often difficult to understand and tolerate a patient's denial. The one who denies arouses contempt and ill-will. It is, therefore, important to emphasize the tension as well as the link between acceptance and denial. A penetrating analysis by Weisman (1972) provides a valuable foundation here (see p. 235).

Denial and acceptance, to some extent, match the expectations of others and are determined by the relationships with persons who are key figures for the patient. In any given situation, every patient balances on a scale between acceptance and denial. Fluctuations have to do not only with the psychological equipment of the patient and the process of dying but also with the person who happens to be communicating with him. Sudden changes along this dimension are often a reliable indication that something crucial is happening in the terminal process.

The Right to Know and to Not Want to Know

This is not the place to discuss the complex problem of whether, when and how the patient should be informed about the diagnosis and prognosis (Glaser, 1966; Koenig, 1969; Hinton, 1966; Waitzkin & Stoeckle, 1972; McIntosh, 1974). A vast amount has been written on the subject, but many of the arguments are subjective.

In the terminal stage the problem of disclosure regarding the patient's prognosis seldom arises. The patient is partly or wholly aware, subconsciously or consciously, that the end is approaching. He has this knowledge because he is dying and this is a psychological process. But his awareness by no means implies a wish to discuss the matter with just anyone. This will depend on whether he is sure that the other person knows how he views the threatening reality. He may want to know some things but not others; consequently, he fears the person he is talking with. The therapist must carefully analyze what is best for the patient and convey this insight to him.

It is often said that the patient has a right to know. This may be true but only if he has a corresponding right to not want to know. Otherwise one is committing a psychological violation. A person who wants to be humane must be able to sense what the dying person can bear and wishes to know.

Losses and Gains

A dying person is located entirely on the loss side of this dimension—he is leaving all that he loves, all that means anything to him and he will finally lose himself.

To offset all the losses ahead one can try to construct gains;

if one is sufficiently attuned to the patient, these may counterbalance the pain and anxiety, at least for a time. What can be given most immediately is oneself, that is, one's support as a person, by being available, coming spontaneously and really participating. It may be a gain for the patient to be accepted as a friend and perceive that the therapist finds the contact meaningful. It may also be a gain to be able to talk for the first time about a humiliation, a past crime, a forbidden attraction—and to be able to talk about this without being judged. It may be a gain if a reunion can be arranged, through the therapist, with a person one has loved but lost, a child or a close friend whom one has not seen for a long time.

The losses are many and their significance varies. It is important to be able to talk about them and to find that there is someone who understands and will remember. The distress of the dying person may be eased by the knowledge that someone appreciates and perhaps admires the way in which he bears his losses.

Hope and Despair

Hope is a somewhat ambiguous concept. It is often said of dying patients that one should not deprive them of hope. Persons who are dying, however, seldom express a hope of survival, of being saved by a miracle. They know they are dying.

The psychological concept of hope (Stotland, 1969) is not simply a naive belief in the impossible. It is considered by Erikson (1964) to be one of the vital values or "virtues" in life: "Hope is the enduring belief in the attainability of fervent wishes." Hope rests on a sense of and a confidence in being welcome and wanted. Hope looks to the future and has a positive, affective glow (Kastenbaum & Kastenbaum, 1971). The will to live is related to hope but hope is an intrapsychic state, while the will to live (and the desire to die) has more to do with action.

A complete absence of hope can lead to despair and make a person dangerously vulnerable. Dying persons are often somewhere between the extremes of hope and despair and can entertain both simultaneously in relation to different aspects of existence. The therapist must enter into and share these experiences as far as possible without himself despairing utterly or hoping beyond reason.

The Will to Live and the Desire to Die

This pair of opposites is related to hope and despair. Both the will to live and the desire to die are often mentioned by hospital staff in connection with dying patients. The psychological realities behind these phenomena are little understood and would certainly be worth investigating more closely.

Doctors' assessments of patients' will to live and wish to die have been studied by Kastenbaum (1965) and Kastenbaum and Kastenbaum (1971), who found that every doctor considered that "his" patients had a more pronounced will to live than other patients. The study was undertaken in a large geriatric hospital where the mortality could be predicted. Patients assessed as wishing to die did, in fact, die earlier than others. It has not yet been possible to identify the criteria which doctors use in their assessments.

The tension between a will to live and a wish to die raises other questions, such as our innermost attitude toward death in general (non-existence) and to our own death. As a rule, this attitude seems to be ambivalent. We often do not want to die but sometimes perhaps we do, depending on internal and external factors. This ambivalence may change during our life. Persons who are severely ill may have many reasons for not wanting to live any longer.

If one is able to be receptive and listen, this ambivalence may become apparent in a dying person. Regardless of whether he speaks or actually does something about it, the dying person may desire death. Death may be tempting and it may be the patient's hope. A combination of anxiety and longing is common in relation to death. If the therapist can bear to share or take part in this, he or she may gain an insight into hidden parts of the psyche. Other questions may arise when the dying person's wish to die takes an active form or becomes a demand for action on our part, i.e. suicide or euthanasia (see pp. 147-151).

Revolt and Submission

While dying a patient expresses his or her feelings in various ways—in words, facial expressions and gestures, as well as through symptoms such as trembling, sweating and difficulty in breathing—to convey anxiety or depression, tension or agitation, hopelessness and many other affective states. One cannot tell whether the silent patient who passively accepts hospital routines is having a more difficult time than the one who reacts violently, living out strong feelings. It is often our preconceptions or prejudices which lie behind the view that the former's situation is relatively tolerable and vice versa. Only a close relationship will reveal whether the silent, submissive patient is, in fact, struggling with deep anxiety and unbearable solitude.

We encounter a scale of reactions from revolt to submission and often have difficulty in finding a balanced response along this dimension. Dying persons who revolt too violently are asked by most people, often including those nearest them, to calm down. If, instead, the patients submit to fate and wait silently for the inevitable, the relatives or staff comment and even tell them that they are giving up too easily.

We are not good at tolerating the behavior of others, especially if—as in the case of a dying person—it arouses our anxiety. We become annoyed and irritated; we readily increase the dose of morphine or soporific still more, just to avoid hearing or seeing. But if one can get to know the person who is dying, it is possible to find an adequate psychological response to his reactions, indicating that one understands him and is on his side. The process of dying is inescapable and the individuality of the patient should be emphasized by permitting him to react as his personality requires.

Identity and Dissolution

During dying identity disintegrates. As this process oscillates, there may be a return to earlier psychological phases and behavior may change accordingly. Still, the process goes implacably towards dissolution. To witness all this is a tragic experience. One can definitely contribute to a feeling of security in the patient if in friendship time and effort have been spent on getting to know and understand the patient's identity in every way. It is comforting if a person who is familiar with the patient can sit by his side in a calm, natural manner. That person will gradually fade into a shadow, a face, a pair of eyes or a familiar voice, but by maintaining the identity of the patient as it were from outside, he generates a sense of security.

Restitution and Regression

This dimension is closely related to the previous one. Its various phases have been described by Weisman (1972). As regression approaches its peak, it becomes increasingly difficult to find one's way in the patient's world. We often regard his talk as psychotic and understand less and less of what he experiences. In this dimension, too, the pendulum swings and the condition of the dying person fluctuates until he becomes confused, slips into unconsciousness and dies.

Security and Insecurity

This dimension is represented in several ways in all those mentioned above, just as they are interwoven to varying extents depending on the particular situation. Security means different things to different people. Dying persons often ask whether I have been present at a death-bed before; on hearing that I have, they comment that it feels comforting. There may be several reasons for this. Having gone through it before implies that one can take it and will not try to escape. In other words, I can stand being present all the time with them, too. Many have asked: "You won't abandon me, will you?"

Many persons are afraid of doing the wrong thing, of dying "unsuitably" or breaking down. One can never be certain what people will say about someone, how he will be remembered, until he has died. The patient finds it reassuring that someone who has gotten to know him and learned to understand and appreciate him will be present and in a sense protect him, besides preserving a favorable picture when he is dead. Such thoughts have been voiced when patients have asked me to remember them. They have obviously found it comforting to know that I really mean what I say when I promise to remember them.

Dignity and Humiliation

To be dying is humiliating. The patient is sick, emaciated, possibly plagued by pain, sweaty, ill-smelling, pathetic, cries easily and begs for help. He is troubled at night and sleeps during the day. Not everyone dies like this but many do. We ensure that everything is done to make things more bearable for them, but we must also accept them as they are without shying away.

In recent years it has become comon to talk about "death with dignity" or a "dignified death." There is a risk of these terms being used as a norm for how people should die (Ramsey, 1974). A preconceived standard for dying must not be urged or forced upon others. Even if this is unintentional, it almost amounts to subjection. Only the dying person knows how he shall die in order to do so with dignity. What kind of death a doctor, clergyman or relative considers dignified is completely irrelevant. If the patient himself experiences his dying as undignified, much can be done by a warm, engaged therapist with psychological insight.

Dying is frequently painful, solitary and unattractive. Consequently, I am skeptical about persons who, after spending time with a dying person, say that they had such "beautiful talks." The dying person and the therapist both contribute something and both benefit from a sincere dialogue. Talks that are described as "beautiful" or "good" would seem to cater more for the need of the therapist than for the person who is dying.

During the process of dying the dignified and the undignified, the ugly and the beautiful, are extremely close to each other.

Living and Dying

This is a self-evident dimension, a component of all the others which constantly confronts the dying person. It is said that people die a little all through life. A patient who is dying does so rapidly and on many levels. But at the same time he is alive and must be treated as a living person up to the end. The therapist must continuously ascertain the patient's condition, his capacity and the course of the process. To lose certain functions and abilities is humiliating, anxiety-promoting and painful. One must, therefore, take advantage of the abilities that remain. At each moment and in every situation the dying person should be allowed and encouraged to function as fully as possible. The life he is still living should be respected and intensified, instead of letting him die a little in advance. By understanding and practicing this, one also makes it easier for the dying person to accept the assistance he may need as abilities decline.

Our primary task is to allow the dying person to live until he dies.

Part II
THE METHOD

Chapter 3

Characteristics of the Method

As already mentioned, the psychological care of dying persons described in this book has, for the sake of brevity, been termed a "method," although it would be more appropriate to regard it as a practical, clinical application of an approach or an ideology of care (Feigenberg, 1975b).

The method is a means of establishing close personal contact with a cancer patient who is terminally ill in an oncological clinic, with regular contacts until death intervenes. In order to focus on the psychological needs of the dying person, I deliberately confine myself to the patient and exclude all forms of contact with relatives and the regular nursing staff. I have typically only one orientation session with the primary relatives of the patient, in which the aim and nature of my approach are made clear to them. I limit my contacts to the patient alone and attempt to become his personal, confidential doctor. In this way—in response to the special situation the patient is experiencing—I create a very special psychological setting in which a friendship is established.

The ideas behind this approach and the content of the psychological contact can be summarized under the following headings.

- *Psychological nearness.* The method aims at intensified psychological contact between patient and therapist. In other words, as the contact develops, both parties should become so confident in each other that they can drop, to a great extent, the resistance and reserve that always exist between people.

A dying person, moreover, always has conflicts, problems and questions that are troublesome to bear alone, at the same time as he or she knows that they will generate unrest, anxiety or aversion in a person who has to share them. Under these circumstances, maximal psychological nearness and as open a relationship as possible are essential if both the patient and the therapist are to experience their contact as meaningful.

- *Dialogue.* The patient must feel that he really can bring up his innermost thoughts, questions and fears and that he will be met with a response—that these matters can be aired and discussed on an equal footing. The communication should be as open as possible, verbally and nonverbally. Right from the start a clear promise is given that nothing that is important and personal for the dying individual will ever be revealed or discussed with others. By excluding all forms of communication (apart from the single orientation) between therapist and relatives, one emphasizes the personal nature of the contact with the patient and the special situation, besides making it easier for the dying person to bring up topics that are important for him emotionally.

- *New friend.* The relation between patient and therapist is expressed here in two words, each with an important psychological content. The relationship is *new,* i.e., the severely ill patient encounters a person for whom he can hardly have either favorable or unfavorable feelings. Furthermore, a new relationship is established at a time when most people under such circumstances are avoided and let down by more and more of their circle. The term *friend* applies to the psychological side of a personal contact which both persons experience as important and meaningful. They become increasingly significant for each other and an emotional relationship develops. The completely exclusive contact means that the dying person transfers many of his feelings and conflicts to the therapist and that the latter in turn reacts to this. The phenomena that are known in dynamic theory as transference and countertransference become central and intense in psychological relationships with dying persons.

The contact established can be called a friendship contract if one accepts a certain limitation on the usual meaning of friendship. Here it is restricted to the special setting and to the psychological aspects.

● *The relatives.* The method described here in no way aims to shut off the relatives from the dying person. On the contrary, they should meet and communicate with the patient according to their wish and need. In connection with my informative session with the relatives, I may refer them to an appropriate professional if need be. At the same time, the dying person harbors conflicts, questions or problems that he either cannot or does not wish to discuss with relatives, either because he wishes to spare them or because it might irritate, annoy or repel them. A completely private contact with an outsider can absorb many of the questions that arise while dying and which might cause tension with relatives. The kind of psychological nearness which a therapist can provide is thus different from that which a family can give.

Chapter 4

The Patients

This book confines itself to work I have done as a psychiatrist at Radiumhemmet in the years 1968 to 1975. In this period I met approximately 170 patients who were dying or had a fatal illness. Of all the 800 or so patients who were referred to me during these years, the proportion who were terminally ill rose from about 10 percent in 1968 to almost 30 percent in 1975. The 170 patients all received some form of psychological terminal care. The types of care provided were determined by many factors, such as the current somatic situation, the patient's personality and pattern of reactions, the staff's attitude to the patient, the latter's contacts with relatives, etc. This care was often given over a considerable period of time; also, I have often cared for relatives as well as the patient. In certain cases I have considered there were indications for the special form of terminal care that is described here. The deliberations that lead up to such a decision will be discussed later.

THE 38 PATIENTS

The material on which this account is based consists of case histories of 38 patients whom I managed in the period from October 1968 to November 1975 in accordance with my method. Data—diagnoses, sex, age, reasons for referral and so on—on these patients are given in Appendix II (p. 254).

Several of these 38 patients were referred to me because they were dying, but I had been in touch with a fair number of them long before they became so ill as to need terminal care. Appendix II lists the original reason for referral and the approximate interval between my initial contact with the patient and the time when terminal care was called for. Only four referrals expressly asked for "terminal care" and another 10 were clearly aimed at such treatment without saying so explicitly. Almost half of the patients (18) were referred to me more than three months before our terminal contact started. Before they became terminally ill I had been in touch with four of these for less than six months, with seven for between six and twelve months, and with another seven for more than one year.

Of the 38 patients, I consider that 14 were referred in what can best be described as the preterminal phase, i.e., at a time when they did not perceive themselves in the psychological sense as dying but felt that they were passing from a state of being severely ill to something still more threatening. In this phase it was possible to plan psychological terminal care meaningfully with a patient whose condition was not unduly poor.

In three cases it must be said that the referrals came too late from the psychological-psychiatric point of view. These patients had been terminally ill for some time when some event suddenly changed their situation or increased the strain on the staff. A relative or someone else, for instance, might suddenly and unexpectedly collapse under the burden of assisting the dying person. In some cases my contact with the patient started late—or at least later than would have been desirable—because he or she at first rejected a proposed referral to a psychiatrist. After a time perhaps the progress of the disease or a change in the psychological situation caused the patient to reconsider the matter and ask for referral.

The duration of the terminal stage in these 38 patients varied considerably, ranging from a couple of weeks to more than a year.

Appendix II also lists the number of sessions during the course of terminal care and an approximate estimate of the total time spent in this way with the patient, including the contacts with relatives before the work with the patient started. This time covers only the sessions themselves.

ASSEMBLING THE MATERIAL

Case records. As in all other work with patients I have kept the usual psychiatric records on the 38 persons considered here. The present report is based on these records. My psychiatric records contain specific data on the occasion for talks, drugs prescribed and other facts. I usually include a short account of the psychodynamic process between the patient and myself and the content of the patient's conversation. Most of what the patient really wanted to discuss with me personally, as well as matters which involved conflicts or tension, have been noted only sparsely. On the other hand, I usually summarize a session immediately afterwards in such a way that the notes remind me of the essential theme. But I never make notes during the course of a talk, partly because this would tend to increase a patient's reservation and partly because I would not then be able to concentrate entirely on listening and observing.

Memory images. The questions and problems that have been mentioned or discussed during each contact with a dying person have etched themselves into my memory just because the person was dying. This applied in particular to the 38 patients considered here, as my contact with them was so special. I am emphatically clear about what passed between the patient and myself and this is supported, moreover, by the information in the case reports. It should be noted that all my contacts with dying patients, including those reported here, were undertaken solely with the purpose of providing adequate psychological terminal care. It was not until the contact with the most recent patient in this group had been concluded that the idea arose of publishing my experiences, discussing the patients and describing the method. Therefore, there was never any question of arranging independent observations or audiovisual aids.

This account accordingly relies to some extent on memory, which can be viewed in different ways as a source of error. The account will be influenced by my subjective feelings, my anxiety and my defenses. Perhaps the experience of talking with dying patients has helped to reduce this source of error. In my contacts with four of the patients, moreover, I received supervision from a psychoanalyst.

The important point, however, is not so much that a source of error exists as that one is aware of its existence. In all research or scientific systematizing there is a risk that the results may be influenced by the researcher's own personality, his attitudes and experiences. This risk is, of course, particularly marked in contacts with the dying. While it would clearly have been desirable to check this source of error, it is difficult to see how such a study could be prevented from conflicting with the aim of my approach (see pp. 187-191).

PROFESSIONAL SECRECY

It goes without saying that as a doctor I am under an obligation to observe professional secrecy. This concerns not only my patients but also their relatives and the hospital staff. Details and specifics have been avoided in order to prevent anyone from being able to recognize the patients. Much the same applies to references which a relative might recognize and be depressed or wounded by. It should be remembered, moreover, that what I relate derives from several contacts with 38 different patients and I have consistently made changes to prevent relatives from recognizing the patient in question. As this account includes effects of the method on those involved in caring for the patients, the behavior and emotional reactions of the staff are described and commented on, too. While some of this information may be regarded as appreciative and favorable, there are also details which are critical and emotionally revealing. Since I never mention departments or wards by name and there is (unfortunately) a high turnover of doctors and nurses, identification is hardly possible.

Chapter 5

Five Case Histories

I have chosen five of my 38 patients as case histories. They will be referred to as patients A, B, C, D, and E. These five patients represent a variety of situations; they have been selected to illustrate different questions and conflicts and some of the courses that dying may follow. I have included both sexes as well as different ages and different types of cancer. But these five cases have not been selected because they were particularly dramatic or in any sense unique. In my opinion, all deaths are equally dramatic and unique if one is sufficiently close to the person concerned. It is only from a distance and with a preconceived opinion that one can regard the death of an old patient with a heart complaint at a nursing home as less dramatic than that of a young drug addict, or the death of an aged widow as of less significance than that of a young mother.

These case histories can awaken very different reactions in the reader. They also illustrate how multifarious death can be.

The case histories are not intended to be complete. On the contrary, essential aspects have been left out deliberately, in keeping with the principles of my method. Neither are they intended to be psychiatric records. The purpose is not to present the structure of the patient's personality, the psychodynam-

43

ics as such, or other components of a psychiatric exploration
of a particular person's symptomatology or morbidity. The
aim is to underline the aspects that are specific for terminal
care and to give a coherent picture of a person's life up to
death.

I have decided *not to comment* on these case histories. This
decision has to do both with my view of dynamic psychology
and with the process of dying. Each word that is uttered and
all that happens are significant and could be commented on
and explained. During the process of dying, moreover, everything that passes relates to earlier events, besides having a
meaning in the immediate situation and links to what the patient hopes and fears will happen. No less important is everything that does not get said or discussed. If all this were to be
presented in order to convey relevant psychological aspects,
one could easily devote a whole book to each patient. I deliberately present these cases for interpretation in keeping
with the reader's personality and psychological-psychiatric
orientation.

These descriptions of patients must also be discussed from
another point of view. My emphasis on the personal, private
nature of the relationship with the dying person may seem
to be contradicted by this presentation of specific cases. I am
convinced, however, that this does not constitute a breach of
my promise to the patient not to disclose anything of a personal nature that has passed between us.

These accounts have been compiled, as already mentioned,
to depict my approach to care of the dying. They are not a
recapitulation of all the questions, problems, conflicts and private or inflammable topics that arose during our talks. I have
excluded anything which seems to belong to the patient's personal, sensitive sphere, as well as everything which we both
knew belonged solely to our dialogue. As a rule, these have
been matters which are of minor importance for an under-

standing of the patient as an individual. While adhering strictly to my agreement with the patient, I have endeavored to recount matters that help one to understand the process. The terminal situation has a particular feature that emerges quite clearly when an open, close relationship is established with a dying person. Both persons are aware of what is sensitive and crucial and of what one shares because both feel secure in the relationship.

In each of the five cases presented here, the closest relative has given me personal, explicit permission to publish the case history and has also been given the manuscript to read. I had planned to include a sixth history but have not done so because the nearest relative did not reply to my letter. There are many conceivable reasons for this and rather than run the risk of applying pressure I refrained from getting in touch in person.

It must have been painful for the relatives to meet me once again, at my request, to read through the manuscript and talk about these case histories. Their positive response meant a great deal to me, offsetting the doubt and anxiety I felt about using these histories here. I should like to say how genuinely grateful I am to them.

PATIENT A

Patient A was a boy of 16 with a metastasing osteogenic sarcoma who had been treated at Radiumhemmet for quite some time before our first meeting. I had already heard a good deal about him. Various members of the staff had said that he was young and intelligent and that they were charmed by him but shaken by his plight. Someone mentioned that he came from a foreign country, having been born in Eastern Europe, but now lived with his parents in Sweden. On one occasion a nurse remarked in a somewhat irritated manner that he occupied a private room, had long hair and kept a guitar in one corner. Clearly he represented a fairly considerable burden for the staff.

I received a note of referral, citing the severe disease and the patient's anxiety but with no indication of the reasons for consulting me or why this should be done just then. Not knowing whether the patient wished to meet a psychiatrist or had even been told that he would do so, I inquired at the ward and received an irritated and somewhat embarrassed reply. It turned out that the patient had not been asked and that the referral had been issued by a house physician partly because some of the staff found A very trying. Therefore, instead of arranging an appointment, I requested that the patient be consulted first about the idea of meeting the psychiatrist at Radiumhemmet.

From the records I learned that A had an osteogenic sarcoma in the left knee. The leg had been amputated a year ago, followed by radiation therapy. For some time he used crutches, then a prothesis. For a while he was able to live at home, but lung metastases were detected only four months after the amputation, whereupon the patient was admitted to Radiumhemmet for increasingly long periods. Finally, the decision was made to care for him there until the end.

One day I happened to see the patient in a corridor, though at a distance and from behind. It was a bizarre sight—emaciated, wearing a long white hospital tunic, this long-haired 16-year-old was swinging down the corridor on his crutches towards the lavatory.

When asked at my request whether he wanted to meet the house psychiatrist, he replied that the psychiatrist could "go to hell and stay there." The same applied to any social worker and all "that lot." He had met their type before and had had enough.

Early one morning two weeks later, however, I received a call from the ward asking me to come at once to meet the boy, who now wanted this himself. While at home over the weekend he had had an attack of coughing with difficulty in breathing and symptoms of suffocation. Both he and the parents were very frightened by this and took an ambulance to the hospital. On Monday morning he said to the ward nurse; "Let me meet the one you spoke about." I asked the nurse to tell him that I would be there at a particular time that day. At exactly the appointed hour I knocked on the door of his room. Receiving no reply, I entered and closed the door behind me. In the middle of the floor was a hospital bed, in one corner the guitar I had heard of. Art books and drawings were strewn over the table and chairs; other drawings had been fastened to the walls with tape. But although there were plenty of things in the room, there was no person to be seen. I sat down on the empty chair next to the bed, on which I suspected that he lay outstretched with the blanket over his head, trying to make himself as invisible as possible. After a while, I said, "Now I think you should look up." The blanket moved, part of a face appeared and a frightened eye regarded me. This attempt to hide from it all expressed more clearly than any words the patient's anxiety about our meeting.

I said, "Look, you're going to have to sit up properly if we are to talk with each other." Gradually he moved up in the bed, adjusted the pillow and looked at me anxiously. "Hello," I said, to indicate that our talk had not started until now, and added, "I think we should be on christian-name terms; it seems simplest to me. What do you say?" He nodded a little nonchalantly and apparently found it okay.

I then said that I had gotten the impression he was having a hard time and seemed uneasy. I suggested we should try to talk about it. The boy was silent a moment and then said: "Do you believe in flying saucers?" I replied that I was not certain that belief was the right word—flying saucers are hardly a religion. But if he meant that what people call flying saucers are vehicles from other planets, then frankly I didn't believe it. But not knowing much about flying saucers, I would like to hear more. I added, "What do you think about flying saucers?" After another short silence, he said, "Do you believe in a life after death?" I replied that this really was a question of belief and that I personally do not believe in a life after death. The idea of life after death, however, is important and complex, and worth talking about. So I said, "What do you believe?" Still no answer, just another question, "Do you believe in Freud?" To this I replied that Freud is not someone one needs to believe or not believe in and added, "Flying saucers, God and Freud—that's rather an odd company." But if he were asking whether I considered that Freud was an outstanding person, my answer would be that many of his ideas were important, much of what he had said was sound, other parts less so. If Freud were still alive, he would presumably alter parts of what he had written and work on other parts until they became still more valuable.

This ended his cross-examination of me about "belief" and in a somewhat disdainful, somewhat hesitant voice the boy said, "I'm rather frightened. What can you do about that?" I replied that perhaps I could be of some assistance with just that. I explained that it might help if we could really talk with each other about how he was feeling, what it was like to be as ill as he was and what he was frightened of, besides going into his life at home, his relationship to his parents, in school, to doctors and nurses at the hospital, his plans for the future and many other things. I added, "You may need someone with whom you can talk about such things and I'm willing to be this person, but whoever does this must be yours alone." He looked questioningly at me and said, "What do you mean?" I replied, "I mean a person with whom you can talk about whatever you want, who knows psychology and is absolutely certain not to discuss you with nurses, doctors or your parents. What you tell me in the future is no one's concern, at least not the things that are important for you." After a somewhat longer silence, the boy looked at me squarely and said, "God damn!"

He then asked how I thought his parents would react. I replied that I would have to talk to them first and asked him to tell them what I had said and to get in touch with me. And so I ended our first talk by promising to come back as soon as I had seen his parents.

The father phoned next morning and we made an appointment that suited the parents and me and gave us plenty of time. When the parents arrived, they were clearly tense. They spoke Swedish well, though with a definite accent, and seemed to have settled down in this country. Our talk started with the mother asking for my opinion about the boy and expressing some expectation that perhaps I would give them a little hope or suggest a new form of treatment that might help their son. I took this opportunity to discuss with them—calmly and at length but discreetly—what the doctors had already told them repeatedly about their son's situation. I indicated that while I understood their despair, I was unable to offer any hope. I considered it essential that at this juncture we should establish together that there was little hope of saving the boy. The mother cried uncontrollably, while the father appeared more collected and tried to remain calm. He explained that he had recently lost other persons who were near to him in his native country and that his faith helped him. I tried to convey my sympathy for them and asked whether they had anyone who could help and support them. A doctor attached to the company where the mother worked knew about the situation and was prepared to help them when they so wished.

I then emphasized that in order to be of use to the boy I would have to devote myself as a psychiatrist entirely to him. I described my particular approach and mentioned the burden which this might impose on them. I also made it clear that after this it would not be possible for us to meet or exchange views.

I had observed the parents during our talk. The mother was more emotional and displayed her grief openly, while the father was more correct and controlled. There was also an air of separation about them; they had placed the two available chairs rather far apart and there seemed to be an emotional distance between them.

The parents then told me a little about their son. He was their only child, born in their native country. He came to Sweden at the age of five, having previously lived for considerable periods with his maternal grandmother. Apparently, the parents had moved to Sweden earlier and waited before bringing over the boy. The parents talked to each other in their native tongue and managed quite well otherwise with Swedish, whereas the son now spoke and wrote Swedish perfectly and, according to the parents, had forgotten his mother tongue. They related that he was often displeased with them for not being sufficiently Swedish, correcting their speech or their manner. They were also at pains to say how attached they were to him, as well as how intelligent and successful he was. Teachers and classmates appreciated him greatly and the parents had been told that much was expected of their son.

A few days after this talk I sent a message to the boy to say that I would call on him at a certain time. When I arrived, he sat up in bed and said, "Well?", adding that he had wondered how the talk with his parents had gone. When I asked whether he had not seen his parents in the meantime and learned about our talk, he confirmed that he had. We then agreed between us that the parents had both understood and accepted the form of contact between him and myself which I had mentioned earlier. This confirmed our agreement and initiated the real contact.

One of my first concerns was to ease his pain, which was considerable, as he had metastases as well as tumor growth in the amputated bone. I wanted to do everything in my power to keep him free from pain and we had a thorough discussion about how long he was helped by the drugs he was taking and whether the doses were large enough. We agreed on a plan of action for the next few days, to be revised jointly if necessary. I pointed out that when prescribing pain-killing drugs I would have to depart from our agreement insofar as the nurses needed to know what we had planned. But nothing else about him would be mentioned between me and the staff.

There then followed a period during which he obviously tested me in various ways, both as a person and regarding the special relationship I had described. I learned subsequently that during the initial phase of our contact he sometimes put questions to the nurses and assistants in such a way that it was clear that he wished to see whether I was keeping my word.

When I asked him about the books that were spread about the room, he brightened up and replied that they were books on art, in which he was very interested. Then he said, somewhat abruptly and defiantly, "What do you think of Dali?" I gave him a thoughtful answer and it was clear that I had passed a test. He then began to talk about his hopes of training to be an artist, a theme to which we returned several times after that.

In the sessions that followed, he talked a bit about his childhood, the situation at home and his other interests. On one occasion, when we had been talking for a while, he said, "Oh, now the pain's starting again." As he had been given an injection fairly recently, I asked what he thought we should do. He answered that when he had pains between injections he usually took a couple of pills. When I asked where they were he said, "Over there," pointing to a table. So I fetched them, poured out some water and gave it to him. Having swallowed the pills, he smiled somewhat shamefacedly: "You see, this was mostly a test—I wanted to see whether I could get a white-haired senior doctor to fetch some pills for me." I replied that I had realized this and added that I could probably endure it, whereupon he smiled and was very pleased when I smiled in return.

It was also at this time that the father phoned me one morning. When I answered he gave his name, apologized for disturbing me and explained that there was something he wished to discuss. I reminded him of our agreement but also said it was understandable if he had very important matters that he felt he wanted to discuss just with me. I also explained that I did not feel like simply replacing the receiver and suggested that we should conclude the conversation but that naturally I would tell the boy that his father had phoned, what we had talked about and so on. Under these circumstances the father let the matter rest. He had been aware of our agreement but had not quite believed that it was to be taken so literally.

I then went straight up to A and told him that his father had phoned. The boy looked tired but he smiled slightly and said, "Yes, I'm not surprised." Seeing a question in my face he added, "There was trouble here with the night nurse. Dad stayed late and when it was time for the next injection on the program, the nurse had disappeared. Dad hurried away to look for her and when he finally found her there was trouble; I don't quite know who said what." Having heard this I asked the boy what he thought we should do and he replied, "Nothing, I can handle the old witch. Don't worry about it—it's possible that Dad overdid it a bit, too."

Keeping the patient free from pain was not easy. There were metastases in the skeleton and lungs. He often had difficulty in breathing and when he coughed the whole body shook, accentuating the skeletal pains. Nevertheless, our relationship became increasingly secure and we talked about many different things. At one of our first meetings I had announced that in about a month's time I planned to be away for a week. He was completely matter-of-fact on that occasion. I told him it was a study trip to look at psychiatry in an East European country—not the one he came from. On a couple of occasions after that, I again mentioned this trip and repeated that I would be away during a particular week. A kind of mumbled confirmation was the usual answer. When I arrived for our last talk before leaving, he opened with, "I have nothing to talk about with you today. Everything is all right." He then turned his face to the wall and I left. He was hurt that I was leaving but also wished to make it clear that it was he who broke the contact with me and not vice versa.

I had assessed the course of his disease and considered that the trip could be made. Moreover, had I not made the journey having mentioned it earlier, he would have understood that I believed that he had very little time left. During the trip I telephoned the hospital a number of times to hear how he was doing.

On my return I called on him at the first suitable opportunity. He lay facing the wall and appeared not to have heard me open the door and enter the room. I sat down and after a while said, "Hello." After some indistinguishable sounds in reply, I asked how things were and received no response. So I said that in that case I would come back some other time and left. I returned at the end of work, late that afternoon, sat down as usual and said, "Now listen, I can well understand that you are angry or disappointed with me for going away, but I do think we should be able to talk about it like two grown men." To this he replied, "What have you to learn in that bloody country?" At this he turned red in the face, suddenly realizing that he had, in fact, paid me a compliment by indicating that I had no need to go anywhere to learn more. In his annoyance he had conveyed that he liked me and was

pleased with our relationship. At the same time, he managed
to indicate that he disliked the country I had visited. I explained that in my view everyone stands to benefit from traveling and seeing how other people solve, say, medical problems.
Some of the things I had seen were good, others less good. He
picked up the question of whether I had anything to learn in
another country and we discussed psychiatric schools and
theories. He was evidently proud to be able to conduct such a
conversation.

One day in his room I caught sight of some magazines
that were not about art. They seemed technical, written for
young persons and more what one would expect of a 16-year-
old than works about Dali and Picasso. Interested, I asked
what they were about and he said mini racing. My questions
then clearly revealed that I had no idea what a mini racing
car is, or what a competition for such cars involves, or why
people travel all the way to England to attend such a competition. (A had done this with a friend after his leg had been
amputated and before the metastases in the lungs appeared.)

The boy came alive, sat up in bed and asked whether I
wanted to learn about this hobby, which I did. For several
visits after that he taught me what he knew, explaining the
hard business side as well as all the technical marvels. His
mother had to bring a mini racing car to the hospital and at
my next visit there it lay in a great many pieces round the
patient and I helped to assemble it. If he was pleased that
I seemed to know who Dali is and was prepared to talk with
him about Freud, then he was unquestionably still more
pleased to be able to teach a senior physician about mini racing cars.

I asked what else he had done in London besides the races.
"We had fun, went to pubs and had a beer." I then asked what
else they had done. "Nothing," was the reply and I had to be
direct and ask whether he had gone out with girls. I was

told that he had not but that there was a girl here in Stockholm with whom he went out.

We talked about many things during the three months or so that our contact lasted. From learned discussions about art and philosophy we turned more and more to personal problems. He told me about himself, his life, his plans for the future, his parents, school and friends. Our tone became increasingly serious and after a time we both realized that he was speaking about things that he knew would never happen. That was why he wanted to tell me about them.

From various clues it was clear that he had a highly emotional relationship with his mother, about whom he talked very warmly. He related that if she arrived at the hospital with eyes red from weeping he would send her out with strict orders to powder her nose and not cry anymore. On one occasion he said that recently he was "nasty" to people and indicated that at times this included his father.

As the boy deteriorated, becoming paler and suffering worse pains, our contact became increasingly confidential. At this time a doctor who had seen a lot of the patient at an earlier stage of his disease came back after several weeks' holiday. I was sitting with the boy when this doctor appeared on his round. He came up to the bed and was confronted by a boy whose entire appearance witnessed to the rapid progress of the disease. The doctor looked at him, perhaps took his hand and clearly wanted to talk but could find nothing to say. He stood a while at the bed, looked helplessly around and left the room. I found him in the corridor when I left and he excused himself with, "I didn't know what to say." A few weeks had created an unbridgeable gap between a sunburned, rested doctor and a young man marked by death. One can understand the doctor. The patient did not say a word about this event but he, too, understood. He gave me a look immediately afterwards and its meaning was clear, but he had neither the time nor the strength to comment.

I visited him more and more frequently. He became muddled about time, often not remembering that I had been there only a few hours before and reproaching me for not coming more often. At times when I held his hand we talked a bit, at other times he fell asleep instead. I heard later that during this period the patient told his mother, "I'm waiting for someone; there is something I'm waiting for. What can it be?" She had then replied that perhaps he was waiting for Dr. Feigenberg to come, whereupon he nodded and said, "Yes, that's it, that's what I'm waiting for. I want him to come."

My visits now tended to be very brief because that was all he could manage. Consequently, I was well able to perform my daily tasks, simply dropping them for a few minutes now and then. It should be added that just as he asked for me and wanted me to come, so I too needed to visit him. After a few hours doing something else, it was only natural to call by his room.

During the last days of the patient's life, I also spent the nights at Radiumhemmet. Sometimes when I came to him he recognized and nodded, sometimes not. A day or so before he died, I came in several times and on one of the occasions when the parents were there I heard a low conversation between them and the boy. I heard him say something incomprehensible but realized that his parents understood. Seeing my questioning look, they told me that the boy was speaking their native language.

Early one morning he asked the night nurse to call his parents to the hospital. I was told about this, as agreed with the staff, and sat with him until the parents arrived. When the door opened and they entered he raised his head slightly and said, "Congratulations mother!" In desperate despair she ran crying from the room. I learned later that it was, in fact, her birthday. The boy died quietly and calmly that evening. I was present when he died and talked about him afterwards with the parents. On that occasion they held their arms around each other; it was the only time I saw any signs of tenderness between them.

PATIENT B

During my office hours one morning I received a call from a ward, contrary to custom and without receiving a referral, and was asked to come at once. A young woman had been admitted that morning even though there was no effective treatment to offer her. She had an advanced cancer of the sigmoid colon. I was told that the staff really did want to look after the patient even though the ward was full and Radiumhemmet does not usually accept such cases. During her admission the patient had suddenly understood her situation and been seized with acute anxiety, hence this appeal to me to help her without delay.

Soon after, on the ward, I learned that the patient, who was 25 years old, had given birth to her first child six months earlier. After the delivery she had bleeding, fever and abdominal pains but the clinical picture did not match the obstetric complications that were first considered. Despite several operations and treatment, her condition deteriorated; three months after delivery, a biopsy showed that she had an adenocarcinoma, probably originating from the lower part of the colon. Palliative treatment was all that could be given.

She had now declined and weighed 80 pounds; the tumor had broken through the abdominal wall and the skin. The department where she had given birth and been treated ever since had sent her to Radiumhemmet for a consultation. In view of the tragic situation, the case history and the patient's age, it was decided to keep her at Radiumhemmet and attempt some palliation with external radiation, even though it was realized that very little could be done for her at this stage and that any attempt at treatment, even for palliation, was debatable. She had been given very vague, conflicting information at the department of gynecology. Someone had mentioned the word tumor, others had spoken about an inflammation but perhaps also about cell changes. Soon after the patient had been admitted, the head of Radiumhemmet came round together with the doctor who had admitted her. As the ward was at this time more than full and several patients might have to be discharged, the chief physician questioned whether this particular patient should have been admitted. This conveyed to her that there was no cure to be had. She suddenly understood the full implications of her position and reacted with understandable anxiety. This was the reason for calling me. It was generally agreed, however, that for humanitarian reasons she should stay at Radiumhemmet.

I entered the room to find a young, pale, emaciated patient. I sat down beside her and we greeted one another, both finding it natural to use the informal form of address. She was open and easy to talk to, with a lively intellect, but she was tense and her eyes were full of anxiety. She burst out at once: "What is this? They say that I may have a tumor, someone even mentioned cancer, surely that's not possible?" I replied that we certainly ought to have a proper talk about her disease at once but that we would have to take up the subject again when the doctors had examined her thoroughly and knew more about it. I explained that the term cancer covers a wide spectrum of diseases, with many forms of treatment. I pointed out that the staff at Radiumhemmet had seen her for only a few hours and that we were in any event determined to do everything possible for her. I concluded by promising that the radiation treatment would start without delay. At the same time I encouraged her to talk frankly about how she had experienced childbirth and, in particular, the period of illness which had lasted ever since.

The acute anxiety died down to reveal a prudent young woman of sound judgment with a good ability to establish a relationship. I suggested that she should tell me a little about herself. She replied with a warm smile and started by saying that she still felt as though she had just given birth and was very unhappy about seeing so little of the baby boy, whom both parents had been looking forward to having. Her relationship with the boy's father was good; they had known one another for ten years and lived together unmarried. Her mother had died about a year ago. Her father was alive and had frequently visited her at the maternity clinic and would certainly come to Radiumhemmet, too. When B spoke about her father I got the impression that there was something grudging and critical in her attitude toward him.

I ended our first talk by pointing out that of course she was seriously ill, that the treatment would take time, and that her situation away from home created many problems and serious questions for her. I therefore suggested that we try to establish a relationship and asked her to tell her husband that I wished to have a meeting with him. I explained that he would have to agree before I could start such a contact. She answered with some pride that there was not much about her life he did not know but that she would be very grateful if I could help her in this way. She would ask her husband to phone me.

My talk with her husband, who was young, unconventional and obviously concerned about the patient, revealed that he was finding life at home rather hard. He had difficulty in managing some of the work with the baby. He had taken a leave of absence from his job and played the role of a parent unquestioningly but could not deny that he found it rather trying. His own parents looked after the child quite frequently. He was interested in sports and found it heavy going at times to sit at home with the baby while the patient was in the hospital. He also indicated that the patient had a poor relationship with her father. I explained my role and why I could not see him again. He could by all means get in touch with other doctors at Radiumhemmet but in the future I would only be B's doctor. This he understood.

The husband visited the hospital frequently and towards the end a couch was placed in B's room so that he could spend the night there. The patient deteriorated rapidly and was often full of anxiety. When she died she had been at Radiumhemmet for five weeks.

I saw her many times during these weeks. At first I visited her twice a week, then three times, and then still more frequently. When I heard that some new measure had been taken, I dropped in to hear whether it had been painful, whether the injection had helped and so on.

She usually spoke a good deal about herself and her life. One day I found that she had a visitor but he left so quickly that I hardly had time to register his appearance. When I asked who he was she replied, "Oh, just the old man." It emerged that she did not think he was worth much, the reason being that he tended to grumble and complain. B felt that even now, when she was ill, it still seemed as though one should feel most sorry for him. It had been the same in relation to her mother, who was now dead. It had always been father who should be pitied and she always had to comfort him. Yet he gave orders and wanted to rule the family, even now that she and her sister had left home.

It was clear, in spite of this, that B's father meant a good deal to her, so I asked whether she had ever discussed her feelings with him. She had not done so, she said, because it would be too much for him. "What do you suppose would happen?" I asked. "He would die, he would have a heart attack on the spot." To this I commented that it might be worth trying to talk frankly to him now.

We dropped the subject and talked about her husband. Their relationship was warm and frank and she also spoke about their small boy. She cried a little and said it made her unhappy not to see more of him. But she also found it rather trying and tiring when her husband did bring him along (in this particular instance the infant was allowed into the hospital). She said that in fact she tired very quickly when he was there, whereupon she usually handed him back to her husband. After a little while, she could not manage to have the infant in her room and told her husband to take him home and come back alone in the evening.

During our first meetings B told me a good deal about her life, her ambitions and her aspirations. As her condition deteriorated, she spoke less and less about the disease, no longer asking about its nature; she accepted but did not discuss her treatment and did not ask about alternatives. Now and then I discerned negative feelings towards this or that person. Having criticized someone she could smile ironically, as though acknowledging her own attitude.

When I entered the ward a day or so after our conversation about B's father, the nurse gave me a look and asked if I was going to see B. Realizing that something was up but that I could not learn anything from the nurse, I went into the patient's room. She was sitting up in bed, which was unusual, and red patches on her cheeks betrayed her excitement. I sat down quietly and asked what had happened.

"Yes, you see, something odd has happened, I got a father yesterday. He sat here yesterday evening, wringing his hands and snivelling. I don't know what came over me but suddenly I felt so angry with him and started to scold him. I told him exactly how I felt. I don't know how I found the courage. I told him what he had been like to mother and what he is like to me now. I really told him how I felt and actually it was a great relief."

After that, she said, he had cried for a long time but then talked to her for a whole hour while she just listened. He explained all sorts of things that she had never known about: his childhood, when he was poor and had a hard time in many ways; how he had met her mother, who came from a better family that never accepted him. He had felt this and B's mother had in fact been rather spiteful to him, which B had never realized before. His life had also been burdened by financial difficulties. Evidently, the father had been able to unburden himself and on leaving he had put his arms round B, who commented to me that "It was the first time that it felt right to hug Dad. The Dad I hugged was a completely new person."

"And then today," she continued, "there was another thing. He came here early, before they started cleaning, so it must have been before 6 a.m., and I got this envelope with money in it from him. My sister got the same amount when she married. As you know, my husband and I are not properly married but now I got my present. It was Dad's way of showing that he thought well of me. I know I won't be able to enjoy the money but it feels good just the same."

B deteriorated rapidly, developing lung metastases and difficulty in breathing. She was pale, weak, vomited a great deal and was frequently in pain, receiving injections for her pain and Valium to decrease her anxiety. Staff members were something of a problem. A night nurse refused to administer Valium and added that she did not care what Dr. Feigenberg had prescribed; B would not get any more Valium from her no matter what she did. On one occasion another nurse had slammed the patient's door with the message: "My patience is at an end." B's husband confirmed these incidents later, describing them in the same terms as the patient. I do not know what had happened, of course, but one wonders whether the nurse's lack of patience was not, in fact, an indication that she could no longer stand the sight of a gentle, friendly young woman wasting away so rapidly. Typically enough, B asked me not to intervene in these situations as the staff might not allow her husband to spend the night there.

I called on her frequently. In one occasion she told me that her father was now very kind to her husband, taking pains to treat him fairly, which he had not done before. Her father was often there, discussing this and that; they were now able to talk with one another.

Towards the end B found it very difficult to be alone, demanded that her husband should be present and was liable to be aggressive toward both him and the staff.

I made brief visits several times a day; sometimes we exchanged a few words and sometimes said nothing at all, but she usually smiled when I arrived. During the final days she was in much less pain and she died calmly and quietly.

PATIENT C

Patient C was a man of almost 40 who was addicted to alcohol and narcotics for many years. A cough which had grown gradually worse for almost a year turned out to be due to a poorly differentiated cancer of the lung which had spread to mediastinal lymph nodes. It had been decided to administer radiation therapy and cytostatics. I had the impression, from the referral and hearsay, that the staff found the patient frustrating and were influenced by his history of drug addiction and criminality. At the same time, it was clear that they liked him, wanted to help him and had no intention of discharging him to long-term care at the end of the treatment.

At our first meeting, the patient started to talk at once, confessing that he carried on too much. I let him talk and listened to a diffuse account of his illness. Although what he said was knowledgeable and full of detail, it had very little content. After a long time, I tried to apply the brakes and asked him to tell me about himself and how he viewed his situation.

I learned that he was born out of wedlock and had never met his father. His mother married again or, as he put it, "was obliged to marry" a man whom C disliked. They had many children, and C had little to do with them. He started at a new school almost every year. After various odd jobs he went to sea for five years. He was somewhat vague about what happened after that but told me frankly that he had led a very irregular life. He had taken tablets and narcotics for 10-15 years, committed crimes of violence and served several terms in prison. He could not remember a time when he had not abused alcohol.

He had been married for four years and greatly admired his former wife. When his drinking got the upper hand they had divorced, two or three years before his illness began. After a short pause for thought, he added that he had a six-year-old son, who had been adopted, and believed that he had another child. He was not entirely sure of this and regretted not having children whom he felt were really his own and whom he had looked after. He believed that having children would have changed his life.

About his illness, C said that "he was clear how things were" and that he was just "waiting for something to happen." He was obviously in pain and coughed heavily and often. When I asked if anyone had discussed his illness with him, he related an episode from the clinic where the diagnosis had been made. Having heard that smoking and lung cancer were connected, he had asked a doctor whether he might light up and was told, "In your case smoking won't make any difference." He had not dared to ask the doctor about anything else just then.

His abuse of narcotics was now a thing of the past. He had a probation officer whom he really liked and trusted. He asked me himself to get in touch with this person, who was a doctor, and I did so in order to form a picture of the situation. C had very few social contacts and the probation officer was about the only person who was close to him.

During one of our first talks, C indicated that he suffered from pain and that he would very much like to take the type of drugs which he had abused earlier. To resolve this dilemma I sought the advice of a specialist, who considered that we could forget his earlier abuse of morphine and administer such doses as his pain required. It would be inadvisable, on the other hand, to prescribe amphetamine or related drugs, that he had used freely, because these might induce behavior which would make it difficult to care for him at Radiumhemmet. I discussed the matter with the patient and explained that he could not expect to get amphetamine either from me or from his probation officer. I strongly advised him not to procure it in other ways as this would immediately cause trouble on the ward. To my knowledge he never did so.

But he was in great pain. The pharmacy at the hospital supplied a 2 percent morphine solution especially for him, in order to keep down the volume injected, and the doses were prescribed by me. I explained to C at length that I was trying to relieve his pain effectively and that he would have to take morphine. Here, however, I ran into an unusual difficulty. This was a man whose ideas had been ruled for years by drug addiction and who had experienced a form of care where everyone concentrated on lowering the dose and withdrawing the drug. Whatever I said or did he interpreted as an attempt on my part to reduce the dose. My intention was, in fact, the opposite, but I wished to increase the dose at a reasonable pace to suit the nature of the pains. On top of this, he had something of a former addict's moral attitude—

now and then he would refuse a morphine injection, for an hour or perhaps a whole day, in order to show himself or me that he could do without it. This was, in fact, infeasible, not because of addiction but because his pains were so severe.

C arrived late for each of our first three or four talks and he never had the appointment card that each patient usually gets from me at the end of a session. After a time he was able to give open expression to his fear and mistrust of psychiatrists. He had met many over the years. At the same time, he had an almost insatiable need to talk. Having sent word that he did not want to come as arranged because he had nothing to say, he would turn up nevertheless and talk unceasingly about everything under the sun. Instead of suggesting a new appointment at the end of a session, I let C decide when he wanted to come back. This invariably started a miniature drama in front of my eyes as he discussed with himself in words and gestures the dilemma of wanting to return as soon as possible in order to continue our talk at the same time as he wished to postpone it for as long as possible because it was not really necessary.

After some weeks, C became increasingly pale and tired. He perspired a lot and was in great pain. I increased the dose of morphine each week. When it was time for an injection he always asked to see the bottle and check that the syringe was properly drawn. This developed into a detailed, meticulous ritual that was observed because the staff understood and accepted it.

C's schooling had been extremely inadequate and he had never obtained any real education; however, he knew a great deal about many things and had a deep respect for knowledge. His powers of observation were remarkable and he recounted many telling situations from hospital life. He indicated that he was always afraid of people at first; he wanted to have time to get to know them; but what he needed most and always coveted was that people should respect him. Meetings with doctors frightened him and initially he was reserved and on guard. Gradually, our relationship became more open and personal and we developed a sort of language of our own with which we could talk about almost anything. On the ward, C expressed his desire for companionship in various ways. He wanted to know what was the matter with all the other patients so that he could get to know them. He was obviously afraid of death but kept circling round the subject. If he learned that a patient had died in a certain room, he showed a child's fear of going past it—a nurse had to accompany him and hold his hand. He was terrified at the thought that someone may have died in the bed in which he lay. Having shown me too clearly how anxious he was over his own death, it happened that he was afraid I would confirm his fears or "say too much" and drowned me in a shower of words to keep me quiet.

After about a month, he started arriving on time and made a show of placing his card on the table to demonstrate that he had not forgotten it. He became more and more confident and accustomed to speaking openly about himself and his life. He told me that he was religious in his own way and that recently he had started to like people more. He repeated more and more often that Radiumhemmet had become a real home where, for the first time, he felt secure and wanted. He returned several times to his request for amphetamine but readily accepted that I could not or would not prescribe it. His pain increased, particularly from the skeleton, and I stepped up the dose of morphine accordingly.

On one occasion when he mentioned this feeling of belonging to Radiumhemmet, he added a little hesitantly that he would like to know more about me. I did not take him up directly on this, but neither did I dismiss the idea. At our next meeting, having talked about his life, his marriage and the difficulties with his wife, he really let go and demanded that I tell him about myself. I told him to go ahead and ask whatever he liked. He wondered whether I was married and I said that I was. He wanted to know if I was happily married and I confirmed that. He asked whether I had any children and when I confirmed that, too, he exclaimed, "This is sensational!" I asked why he thought so. His reply indicated that he drew satisfaction from it as proof that Radiumhemmet, and I as part of Radiumhemmet, were reliable and harmonious.

After a few more questions, he fell silent, collected himself and suddenly asked, "You have had cancer, haven't you?" Before I could answer, he added that somehow he thought I had, explaining with some embarrassment, "You understand us so well that we assumed you must have had cancer yourself." I told him truthfully that I have not had cancer but that this could happen to me just like anyone else.

C's condition deteriorated rapidly; he became increasingly confused and was given cortisone. He told me he felt the end approaching and related his thoughts about this, concluding the talk by asking whether I would certify that he was fit to hold a driving license. I said that I was willing to do so when the time came. He died shortly afterwards, unfortunately with violent pains and something of a struggle because the doctor on duty did not dare to increase the dose of morphine.

PATIENT D

Patient D, a woman of 50 with a generalized malignant melanoma, was referred to me because she had asked to see a psychiatrist. At our first meeting, she was alternately aggressive and desperate and obviously needed psychiatric assistance. Although under great pressure, she held her distance, speaking about her situation and illness in general terms. As I listened, it became clear that D was an intelligent woman with an academic profession. She was married, with two children. I let her speak freely and soon noticed a clear discrepancy between what she was saying and her desperate situation. Her aggressive outbursts seemed to be a revolt against fate and not aimed at me or the health service.

Towards the end of this first meeting, she suddenly checked herself, started to cry and said: "I can't handle this. I know in my mind that I have a serious illness, I understand that clearly, but I cannot deal with it. I am completely nonplussed and helpless and cannot talk about it with anyone, neither my husband nor anyone else." In a short time we had actually established a good relationship and I indicated that I was willing to support her. I said that I would certainly be available so that she would have someone to talk with openly about her feelings and I proposed that, having talked with her husband, I should confine myself to her.

Some days later I met her husband, a big, powerful man with a shock of dark hair and large gestures. He was clearly tense about our meeting and started talking about his wife even before he sat down. He described her illness, her symptoms and her behavior, emphasizing that she was an extremely ambitious woman, very self-critical and never really satisfied with herself. He also described himself spontaneously as a man who was used to managing and deciding things. He realized that this might not be a good thing but that's how it was. He expected others to do what he said. He believed that perhaps this was why they sometimes quarreled at home. He talked for quite a long time, providing valuable information about his wife but also obtaining some relief from his own predicament. Throughout this lengthy account, he maintained an ironical tone directed against himself.

When this part of our talk was over, I took up his wife's situation, the serious prognosis and how I viewed my task as a psychiatrist. He listened and nodded agreement. Suddenly he bent over the table and started to cry convulsively. I let him be and afterwards he apologized profusely. I explained that he really had nothing to apologize for; it was entirely understandable that he had cried and that he was upset about his wife's plight. When he had assured me that he entirely agreed with the way in which I intended to care for his wife, the meeting ended.

D, who had been discharged from the hospital, came for our second talk two weeks later. She started by telling me about her illness. Two years ago she had noticed a lump in the right groin. Two doctors had both "deceived her" and said it was nothing serious. Almost a year went by before the lump was removed, whereupon she learned that it was a metastasis from a malignant tumor which could not be located. It was then found that the tumor had spread in the abdomen; she had attacks of pain at times and realized that there was a risk of intestinal obstruction. She had been treated with various cytostatics but had a feeling that the doctors did not really believe they would help, although they were very insistent that she should take them.

She then related that her husband had started to lend a hand at home, which she appreciated in a way, though it also made her feel guilty: "It's something that the man of the house should not need to do." Suddenly she broke off and asked whether I had seen a recent television program in which two public figures had discussed life and death in a very personal manner, adding abruptly with great feeling, "Isn't he loathesome?" It turned out that the man, who happened to be Ingmar Bergman, talked far too much about himself; she found it dreadful that he spoke so openly about himself and about his relations with people who were close to him, adding that she felt she was having a much more difficult time than Ingmar Bergman.

In the space of a few minutes, D then related things which she had previously indicated to me only superficially and indirectly. She regarded herself in every way as a failure—as a mother, a wife and at work. She had thought of suicide on several occasions in the course of her life and had been admitted to a psychiatric clinic eight years ago after attempting suicide. Since then she had gone to a psychotherapist for several years but did not feel it helped much. Even now she felt a failure and inadequate, with a longing to get away from it all. She made the dry comment that it was no longer necessary to attempt suicide, it was all going to work out on its own.

Her husband phoned me some days later, sounding very reproachful and aggressive; he considered that my care of his wife was highly unsuitable. I reminded him of our agreement and said that I would talk with his wife about our conversation. He was agitated and I recommended that he, too, should consult a psychiatrist (he had told me earlier that there was one where he worked). To justify his call he told me that his wife was threatening to commit suicide. When I still remained noncommittal, he went on: "She has been cared for very badly, she has a large lump in one armpit and her doctor has told her that it's a metastasis." I then asked whether he thought the doctor should have said it was something else, something harmless. I admitted that one could discuss when and how a patient should be told such a thing but that obviously his wife, who had been informed about her disease and was an intelligent person, knew what it was all about. He agreed but was clearly shaken and in a desperate situation. As I understood his anxiety and we were already in touch in this way, I informed him that I was in contact with his wife, that I knew she had contemplated suicide and had talked with her about this only a few hours before. D had not told him about our talks or the latest meeting.

The next time I saw D I related my conversation with her husband. She listened in silence and said thoughtfully that perhaps her chief problem was not her husband but her own father. She said, "I fought him because he was so domineering. He dominated me and he dominated my mother. At the same time I loved him. I think in a way that I'm responsible for his death and it troubles me." I encouraged her to tell me a little about her parents.

She had grown up in a house by a lake in central Sweden. She was not quite 20 when her mother died of a thrombosis. Her father, a big, colorful, dominating person, was greatly grieved by the death of his wife. One winter's day soon afterwards, D went out onto the ice even though her father had strictly warned her not to. The ice gave way, some neighbors saw her plight and alerted her father, who immediately went out and saved her but was drowned himself. The enormous significance of this event for D became evident during our talk. She had wrestled with the problem of guilt for years and discussed it during her psychotherapy, but it still engaged her 30 years after the event. It also featured, of course, in her thoughts of suicide and partly explained why she said that she welcomed her fatal disease.

Although she was pale, tired and obviously worse at this time, D put a great deal of effort into planning a journey with her husband to Denmark. She wanted them to visit some friends and obviously set great store by this trip. She knew that her tumor was growing and this made her anxious to carry out her plan. As the journey meant so much to her emotionally, I supported her decision. Her husband would drive their station wagon, in which she could travel lying down, and she would have a letter to doctors in Denmark about her disease and conceivable complications. She hoped to be away for at least a month if she was strong enough and we did not fix a date for our next meeting.

One day about a fortnight after D's departure, I met her husband at the hospital entrance and he told me she had been admitted to Radiumhemmet five days earlier. No one had informed me that she had been there for several days. After ten days or so in Denmark, she had felt so down that the visit was broken off and her husband had driven her as fast as possible right across Sweden to Radiumhemmet.

I went up to the ward as soon as I had obtained her husband's assurance that she really wanted to meet me. I explained what had happened and said I was sorry no one had told me she was there. Her poor condition when she arrived had prevented her from getting in touch with me. She was still weak from the strain and in need of further care and additional fluid. I told her that I expected she would improve somewhat soon and we arranged a new meeting in a week's time.

I found her sitting up in bed and strong enough for a longer talk. She said that her thoughts were again circling round her parents. She had arrived at the conclusion that, although she ought not to have gone skating on the ice, perhaps it had not been her fault that her father had drowned.

"When mother died, my father's life came to an end. He showed no interest in anything. He was manager of a small company and did not neglect that. He went to work every day even after mother's death. But he also visited her grave almost daily. It seems he must have had a depression. Then came that day on the ice. I was floundering in the water and he rushed out to rescue me. He needn't have done so; I could have managed perfectly well on my own. I believe there was an element of suicide in it. You don't act like that unless you are dissatisfied with yourself and your life, which I believe father was. I don't believe it was entirely my fault. There was something self-destructive about father, too."

It was the first time that D had dared to pursue the thought that she was by no means to blame for her father's death. In our relationship it was a confirmation of frankness and mutual understanding.

General care and a new course of cytostatics produced a

somatic improvement, whereupon D started to overestimate her resources and deny her illness, even planning to resume work. She relapsed very soon, however, becoming pale, tired and influenced by the drugs. She spoke about her disease again and said she was well aware of the situation. She was now in a ward at Radiumhemmet and we talked frequently. Her matter-of-fact assessment of her hopeless condition was accompanied by frequent signs of irritation over apparently minor details in the hospital routine. She found the nurse's visits with food or medicine at set times very frustrating; she did not like others to decide when and what she would eat. She also objected to the doctors coming and going just as they pleased.

"I have always found it extremely difficult to allow other people to manage and order me about. It feels as though I were a prisoner. And I know that that is what I am, the prisoner of my disease. That's what has put me in this position."

On several occasions D took up her relationship with her husband and told me they had found each other difficult at times. In particular, the periods when she had undergone psychotherapy had been a strain for him, too. Her description of her father suggested that her husband resembled him; in any event, D found them both dominating. It was also clear that she had difficulty in talking about her illness and death with her husband. On one occasion she remarked that he could not bring himself to discuss her illness with her; then, after a short pause for thought, she added that neither could she really bring herself to talk about it with him.

She talked with me about her illness in clear, matter-of-fact terms. She pointed out that there were metastases under the skin on her neck and that new ones were starting to appear. She indicated that it was important for her to be able to talk realistically about her illness and not have it explained away or covered over; at the same time, it was a relief to be able to display irritation about her treatment without hurting me. On this occasion she took up personal, painful questions about what lay ahead for her and those nearest to her and we ended the talk by agreeing to use Christian names in future, indicating that we had become close friends and could talk about essential matters.

In the days that followed, D's distress from her abdominal pains increased and I stepped up the doses of analgesics. One day I met the senior physician on his rounds of the ward and he informed me that D was now "completely out of her senses." She had behaved quite unreasonably and an infusion with narcotics was being planned so that she would not only be free from the pain but also sleep calmly right up to the end. I did not discuss this, particularly as I could not find out in what way she was "out of her senses." I found D dejected and irritated with the nursing staff but almost demonstratively friendly toward me. I let her talk for a long while about herself and toward the end she hinted that she was aware of having irritated the doctors. She was unhappy about it but still angry.

I asked her to tell me what had happened and she related that during his round the senior physician, after a brief greeting, had removed the sheet without any warning and started to examine her abdomen. This had made her so furious that she started waving her arms and screaming. She had lost her temper chiefly because she knew that her abdomen was hard and full of metastases; she felt it several times a day and knew that the tumor had grown. She also knew that there was nothing to do about it and therefore considered that the doctor had other, more important matters to attend to on her behalf instead of humiliating her with meaningless examination.

D was terminally ill but her mind was obviously clear, oriented and full of insight. She had a great deal left to talk about with me and still more with her family. Psychologically, her life was not yet at an end. I was therefore opposed to the idea of an infusion, especially as this seemed to be more for the sake of the doctors than for her. Unless there are very strong reasons, a dying person may not be deprived of the possibility of winding up life or concluding close relationships in a personal way. I therefore got in touch with the senior physician in question and said that I was opposed to a continuous analgesic infusion in this case. He was irritated and said that in that case I would have to accept responsibility for and take over the analgesic treatment until the end; this was beside the point because I had been handling this treatment before this incident.

The next morning I found that the preparations for an infusion had been started, instead of the measure being cancelled. I told D that I did not approve of a continuous infusion and wished instead to change to morphine alone, which I would administer moderately so that she would be clear for part of the day. She felt relieved and agreed with this. In the time that remained, I visited her briefly about twice a day.

At this stage her husband came as often as he could bear to. It was frequently difficult for them both. On the day before she died, they had talked for a while with each other when she suddenly looked up at him and said, "How are we two going to manage this?" He started crying and so did she and nothing was said after that. They held hands and when she had fallen asleep he went home. The next day she died.

That afternoon I met her husband, who was already dressed in black. He came straight up to me and said emphatically, "Thanks." By way of explanation he added that it may or may not have been my doing, but his wife had said to him, "How are we going to manage this?" and it was the first time for many years that anything of the kind had passed between them.

PATIENT E

This patient, with whom I was in touch for almost two years before her death, was a woman of about 60. She had undergone an operation for cancer of the breast almost a year before being referred to me by a doctor at Radiumhemmet. She had been his patient for some time and, appreciating how difficult she found it to change doctors, he had promised to look after her in the future, which he did.

When the patient was referred to me she had skeletal metastases and spinal pain. The doctor asked me to take on the patient and give her psychological support until the end. He considered that she needed it and promised of his own accord to keep me informed about examinations, changes and so on in order that we could give E consistent information and coordinate our measures. He also informed me spontaneously that he knew about my approach and that if and when E became terminally ill, he would avoid communication with me specifically about her personal, private or psychological problems.

My first meeting with E revealed an intelligent, lively, extroverted woman of pleasant appearance. She was a professional person and was quite obviously ambitious and competent. Her illness colored the tone of her conversation but she was able to get outside herself, joking about herself and chaffing me about the part she believed I would play. As we had already gotten on well at this first meeting, I raised the idea of continuing in the way described here, briefly outlining how I concentrated on the patient and excluded all relatives.

She replied at once, "Of course, what else. Good heavens, Doctor, you're not to involve my husband or anyone else if you're going to be my doctor." To which I replied, "That's just what I said, Mrs. E. I believe you need a doctor of your own." At which she laughed and added, "Yes, but on the other hand, there's nothing wrong between me and my husband." So I asked her to tell me and heard that her husband was a senior official and they had a grown-up son. During her disease she had always been able to talk with her husband about everything. Then she added, "I need you, Dr. Feigenberg, for something else and you are not to get in touch with other people behind my back, for then I would have no use for you." We used the formal mode of address in this and in all our future talks.

During our early meetings, she told me a good deal about herself and how she experienced her disease. She was most upset by the need to obtain treatment, including cortisone, for her metastases. She could not bear to be made dependent in this way. Her character was such that she found it detestable to adapt her schedule to the injections and treatment that her illness required. She had been independent and energetic all her life, had always looked after herself and hated being dependent on others.

During the first year of our relationship, E worked full-time, led an active social life and drove her own car to Radiumhemmet. Her prognosis was, as she knew, very poor, but of course she was not dying. At this time I saw her once every two or three weeks to provide support, an opportunity for her to discuss what she wished with me and a chance for me to get to know her.

It was very clear that she found her illness extremely humiliating and knew that her life was threatened. Her marriage was a happy one and her husband supported her to the full, but she was an independent person and wished to spare him as much as possible. "You see, Dr. Feigenberg, it's not good for me to be as ill as I am now. I have, in fact, thought several times of making an end of it but I have come through by myself. My pride tells me to manage everything myself. I have been able to so far and have now dropped those thoughts. I am very fond of my husband and want to spare him."

E related that she found it very difficut at times to deal with people. She met a great many in her profession and was usually able to be as friendly and relaxed as before, but sometimes she was angry and aggressive without being able to understand why.

Medication was something she did not really accept, particularly the cortisone that she now had to take. This had caused her to put on weight. Only about a year before, considering that she weighed too much, she had slimmed energetically and successfully. This was after her operation for breast cancer and her weight loss had not been due to that but to an act of will. She now found it very unpleasant to have to take medicines that caused her to put on weight again. Her concern with her appearance conflicted with her concern to obtain treatment for her disease.

Her doctor and I both realized that she needed to be allowed to decide about her medication, but if we simply said that it was up to her to decide, she became anxious and unhappy: "How should I know whether I require this or not?" On the other hand, if we said that she had to take a particular medicine, she reacted immediately and refused to be ordered about. Being intelligent, she recognized the trap but she also had a sense of humor; so although the situation tormented her, she was able to laugh both at herself and at us.

As she often asked my advice about her medication, it was essential that her somatic doctor and I keep in touch about her attitude toward the current treatment. It was most important that we not give her conflicting information. It turned out that she consulted a book on pharmaceutical preparations in order to learn about the indications for and adverse reactions to the drugs she was taking. It was possible to cooperate with her over treatment, provided one was prepared to give detailed reasons for prescribing a particular medicine—she was extremely hurt if the information was not clear and frank.

E returned now and again to the thoughts of suicide. It happened that she had asked her doctor for a prescription for the sleeping pills she had been using and for no particular reason he ordered a smaller package than usual. When she collected the medicine from the pharmacy, she noticed that there were only 25 tablets instead of the usual 50. This made her so furious that she threw the bottle onto the floor and left. Naturally, she regretted this a couple of minutes later and was obliged to come to me for a new prescription. She was then able to laugh at having thrown away the 25 tablets in her rage, but also mentioned that she had found the situation humiliating.

Although E had difficulty in accepting her disease, she did see her situation fairly clearly. Early on she told me firmly, "Dr. Feigenberg, you may prescribe the medicines I am to have, but I must be able to drive a car." To this I replied, "In that case there won't be much medicine because I don't want you to kill yourself or anyone else in a car accident." When she arrived for one of our next talks she commented sadly, yet in a bantering tone: "Well, I've turned in my car; I've noticed that I really am ill."

Before E came to Radiumhemmet she had had some controversies with doctors at the hospital where she had been operated on. One occasion was immediately after the operation, when she was scorned for not being able to look at her body with one breast removed. Words were exchanged and in the end the senior physician phoned E at home, said that she was unquestionably right and apologized. The next conflict arose with the first local recurrence. She had asked a doctor what it implied and what should be done but he, a religious person, avoided the question and simply replied that the time had come to be reconciled with one's God.

On some occasions she told me that she wanted to break off all treatment. When I replied that she was free to do so, she displayed considerable anxiety but in a sense it also calmed her. Much of our early conversation dealt with the disease and her situation at that time. My task was to let E describe her panic-striken revolt against the captivity imposed by the disease and its treatment and her feeling of impotence when, in spite of her feelings, she could not bring herself to break off the treatment. At the same time, I had to accept and meet her violent outbursts, deep distress and mocking laughter, all of them firmly embedded in her personality.

During the first part of our relationship, it was difficult to start talking about her background, parents and childhood memories. But after several months E herself opened one day by declaring that she would like to spend a long time talking about her youth and the like.

She was the oldest child and had always felt that her parents were disappointed that she was a girl. They had wanted a son and when a boy was born a year or so later they concentrated entirely on him.

Her father was an alcoholic and there had been several suicides in his family. E was warmly and emotionally attached to him but had concealed this as a child because he seemed to be chiefly interested in her brother. Her father was younger than her mother and erotically active, prone to approach any girl he came across. E related, for instance, that a young girl, a distant relative, had lived with them after losing her parents in an accident; she was entirely dependent on her relatives, who employed her in their home. E's father immediately started a relationship with this girl. E's mother discovered this, became frantic and threatened to commit suicide, to which her husband replied that in that case he would do the same. As a result, for several years in her late teens E was worried that something would have happened when she came home from school, that she would find one or perhaps both her parents lying dead on the floor. In this context she also said, "Honestly, my father was quite incredible. He messed about with me, too. When my breasts started to form he was always wanting to feel them."

Her education complete, E escaped from the pressure at home by moving to the north of Sweden, where she met her husband. In later years her mother became very religious and a member of Christian Science, but E, who was not particularly opinionated in such matters, could not share her experience. When her mother died, her father told E that her mother had grieved for her and had died unreconciled. In spite of everything she related about her childhood and family, she indicated that she had loved her parents.

As the disease progressed and cytostatics had to be used, E became increasingly down-hearted, partly because her appearance changed and she lost hair. In time she had to wear a wig and one could detect a change in her features as a result of the hormone therapy. She also developed visible metastases on the skin and this precipitated an appreciable fear of death, which we were able to discuss very thoroughly. She arrived for some appointments and sat completely silent, which I let her do; at other times she talked unceasingly. Once she said, "I'm two persons, the one who runs the house, carries on from day to day, cooks and sits and talks with my husband, and the other who has all these side-effects of cortisone and chemotherapy; I hate and detest that other damned woman, who also exists and is part of me."

E thought of suicide at times but we were able to discuss this openly and agreed that she would phone me if she contemplated putting an end to it all. She did telephone me once from the center of Stockholm, where she had agreed to meet some friends from work. She felt that what she most wanted to do was walk straight out into the traffic. I tried to convey that I understood her intense feeling and that I would not regard it as "bad or wrong" if she followed her impulse. I also suggested, however, that I would phone a pharmacy near her and asked her to collect some tablets, take one of them and then meet her friends as arranged. After that, if she wished, she could call on me at the hospital. On that occasion she turned up. On another she did not, but phoned me later in the day to show there was no need to worry.

During our talks she mentioned having an activity which engaged her. As I had understood that she was slowly closing down her professional life, I wondered what it was. At this she smiled and said she was extremely attached to very old ladies. She had had a couple of clients in their 80s whom she visited or took out, besides cooking and baking for them. Her present concern was a rather irritable, egocentric woman of 90, who clearly terrorized E quite a lot. But E gave me a cheerful, humorous account of all the aggressiveness which the old lady needed to pour out over her. She took it very calmly and easily.

On one occasion I suggested that she ought to devote herself to truly meaningful matters and find time to do the things that gave her personal satisfaction. In reply she exclaimed, "What an idiotic piece of advice to give a grown woman. Are you out of your senses?" And then she left. But next time she said, "Thanks for the good advice. I've actually started to follow it and am doing quite well."

During this period I had been interviewed by a journalist about the emotional impact of cancer and how the care of cancer patients is organized. On the day the interview was published, my secretary informed me that E had phoned to say that she would not be coming anymore—she did not want to risk appearing in tomorrow's paper. After no more than a week, she called back for a new appointment and said when she arrived, "I do really think it's quite excellent that the papers write about cancer and that people begin to understand that one can talk about it—but it still made me very angry.

It all seemed to be about me, even though there was actually nothing about me or any other patients." During a talk E mentioned that, although she was happy to come and discuss things, she often became agitated later at home. I replied that the decision lay with her. She ended the conversation and said at our next meeting, "So you are thinking of abandoning me, Dr. Feigenberg." I asked what she meant and she explained that when I had said that it was up to her to decide whether or not to come, it felt as though I wanted to get rid of her.

Her need for help was struggling, as so often happens, with her desire to manage on her own. Had she been given a fixed appointment once a week or once a month she would undoubtedly have experienced it as coercion and even wanted to stop seeing me. Yet, when I said it was up to her, she felt rejected. I decided to take up this problem and said, "I should like to say once and for all that I really care for you, Mrs E, as you yourself know very well. I like you and I find our meetings very rewarding when we talk about life and death but also when you joke with me and when I criticize you. But you are also my patient and consequently must feel that you come here of your own accord." We then agreed that each time we would jointly decide whether and how soon she wanted to come back. And if she felt unable or unwilling to come one day, she was free not to do so but should keep me informed.

There was a period when E wanted to meet her friends and acquaintances; in a sense she was saying goodbye to them. On one occasion she related that she had arranged to lunch with a man she knew. He took a delight in women and was always very attentive and she thought it would be fun to go out with him. Then she giggled slightly and added, "I must take care not to lift my wig; he'd simply faint."

As the disease progressed, we met more often, now usually

once a week. At times we discussed how E's husband probably experienced her illness, her contact with me and, for instance, the periods when she considered putting an end to it all. She explained that she had talked with her husband about our sessions and had earnestly requested him not to get in touch with me and accordingly trusted him not to. She also made it quite clear that under no circumstances would she tolerate any communication between me and her husband.

She spent short periods at Radiumhemmet and found difficulty in accepting the restrictions and dependence of hospitalization. The first time this happened she felt as though "the world had collapsed." A wise nurse made things easier for her. During a pleural drainage this nurse told her that after a large drainage the patient usually stayed in the hospital but that on this occasion E should just rest a while in the ward and have a cup of coffee. This she did, became acquainted with the staff, glanced into a couple of the rooms and then went home. Next time she herself considered that it would be just as well to spend the night there.

Even when she was staying at Radiumhemmet, we kept to the appointed times and met in my office; only occasionally did I visit her in the ward. Earlier, whenever I was going to be away for some time on holiday, for instance, I had given E the name of another psychiatrist with whom I had an arrangement, but she had never gone to him. Now that she had deteriorated and the summer was approaching, she took up the matter herself and said very firmly, "Yes, Dr. Feigenberg, I really do want you to take a holiday as usual, that's how I want it to be in my case. While you're away I'll take the opportunity and stay in the ward, where I have my ordinary doctor." Before we first met, E had known that the doctors did not expect to cure her and that her time was limited. We had discussed all the emotions which this aroused many times. It did not prevent her from living and being alive. She worked, ran her home and made several journeys abroad. During the latter part of our relationship, it became clear that she was dying. Both she and I and no doubt also her husband and son knew this. There was little means of telling exactly when the transition occurred.. She was certainly aware of it before the rest of us; by means of many subtle changes in the psychological content of our conversation, her mood, the pattern of her movements and so on, she conveyed to me that she was now dying.

During these two years I had experienced the transformation of a vital, extroverted, active woman into a severely emaciated invalid who had great difficulty in breathing. She made her last few visits in a wheelchair, commenting somewhat ironically: "The old girl's seated now." Her husband accompanied her on that occasion; it was the first time I had seen him. The next time she had already changed; her eyes were expressionless and she understood only part of what I said. But she held out her appointment card and said, "I want the next appointment in a week's time—write down the date."

At the time of the next appointment I was met by her husband, in mourning. He said that he had come instead of his wife and assumed that I had been in the country and had not learned from the papers that she had died a few days earlier. I asked him to come in and we had a fairly long talk. Among other things, he said that he quite understood my agreement with his wife and that she had wished there to be no contact between the two of us. He had kept this promise even though he had wanted to phone me on several occasions. He talked about his wife and how much she had meant to him. I thanked him for our talk and told him how much I appreciated having met and known her.

Chapter 6

Choice of Approach

The five case histories in the previous chapter constitute one way to illustrate my approach to care of the dying. Considerations about why and when to use this method, followed by a systematic description of how to establish and accomplish the contact, are other ways.

THE APPROACH TO THE RELATIVES

One of the characteristics of the method is that I choose to concentrate on the patient and exclude the relatives, and this may need some discussion.

The family has been a social institution in our culture since time immemorial and it is natural for us to share the joys as well as the sufferings and sorrows of life with those nearest to us. Since the way in which people react when a serious illness hits a close friend or relative has to do with cultural, social and psychological factors, the pattern varies between countries and within social strata.

Presently, psychodynamic psychiatry is attempting to systematize knowledge and develop models for treating relationships and processes in the family. The practice of including the whole family or some of its members in psychological-psychiatric work has been evolved as one form of treatment.

The occurrence of a fatal illness obviously affects the other members of the patient's family. This problem has been analyzed by several researchers, who have tried to develop models for terminal care with this in mind (Sheldon et al., 1970; Maddison & Raphael, 1972; Baider, 1973; Bermann, 1973; Worby & Babineau, 1974). Most writers involved in care of the dying report that they try to look after the family, too, and include those nearest to the patient in the therapeutic situation. This is, indeed, a welcome development, though it is by no means always clear how much attention and consideration have, in fact, been paid to the patient and the relatives respectively. It should not be thought that I do not agree with the ideas underlying family therapy just because I have developed an exclusively patient-centered approach. In my opinion, family therapy and related models are appropriate and justifiable in many situations, including terminal care.

In special situations, however, I have chosen to screen off the relatives in my contact with the dying person in order to achieve frankness, a close relationship and in an effort to cater to his or her needs and interests. In many situations, it seems to be the only way to make the patient feel free to speak openly about whatever is on his mind. The chief reason for this is that most personal relationships are ambivalent and this is often particularly true of family relationships. These have been rendered complex by the conscious and unconscious conflicts and feelings that form part of a long life, whether or not it has been possible to talk about them. During the process of dying, ambivalent feelings about relatives tend to erupt into conflicts that are difficult to control, confining the dying person to loneliness, feelings of guilt, and pain. It is often a considerable relief to be able to talk openly about this with an outsider, knowing that it will go no further. This quite frequently reduces the affects towards relatives, making it easier for them and the dying person to communicate.

My deliberations about choice of approach are colored by memories from years ago, when I first started to assist dying persons as a psychiatrist at Radiumhemmet. In some cases the patient derived support from the family and it then seemed reasonable to talk with them together. In certain instances, the ambivalent nature of the patient's and relatives' feelings caused the family's problems and conflicts to acquire almost monstrous proportions when they were confronted with approaching death. At times I felt that the only thing to do was keep the relatives away by every means at my disposal, so that the patient might die in peace and quiet. This was hardly humane for the family but the situation was such that it was the only way of doing anything for the patient.

It should also be realized, however, that even warm, strong family ties can constitute a problem when a member of the family is severely ill or dying. Of course, the other members are and want to be at hand to support, assist and comfort. Out of consideration for them, however, the dying person may want to spare them and tries to conceal his grief and despair. The relatives for their part cannot bring themselves to talk about what is really happening and the matters that are truly important to the patient. All their feelings and emotions revolt against looking realistically at the waning strength of the dying person and talking with him about dying and death. The emotional ambivalence among persons who are close to one another and this need to protect one another combine to create a situation where many, but by no means all, practically cease to communicate.

My approach grew out of attempts to analyze these experiences. Studies in thanatology, chiefly those by Eissler (1955) and Rosenthal (1957), confirmed and supported my view of these matters. In most of my subsequent contacts with dying persons where I found reason to exclude the relatives and offer this method, the patient has expressed his satisfaction and appreciation.

> One of the first patients with whom I not only had these viewpoints in mind but also explicitly stated the goal for my work was a woman of 35 (patient no. 6 in Appendix II), whose relationship with her husband and children was warm and harmonious. She was still in a relatively good condition when it was found that her malignant tumor had spread, but she was fully aware of the situation and knew that her time was very limited. She naturally wanted to go on seeing her family as much as possible, but also wished to spare them. It was she who had asked to see a psychiatrist who would provide support in the time that was left. Her contentment was very apparent when I indicated during our very first meeting that I was to be *her* doctor and would not have anything to do with her family. She told me later that my arrangement had made a deep impression on her and made it very much easier for her, in the time that remained, to keep her family relationships on a bearable emotional level and cope with her own feelings.

The patients concerned have interpreted my approach as I intended, namely that I understand their difficulties in connection with relatives and wish to concentrate on their own experiences during the process of dying, emphasizing the frankness and closeness of our relationship. They have indicated that this made it easier for them to bring up old problems, injustices and matters which they believed no one would ever share.

INDICATIONS

Professional psychological terminal care is indicated whenever a dying person needs to talk personally with someone else about the situation. When considering the indications for this method, the first condition is that terminality is involved.

Terminality

The state of dying and of consequently needing terminal care has very little to do with the somatic diagnosis (Feigenberg & Fulton, 1977). Dying is a period in which the individual experiences the threat of death on an emotional level and it ends with the patient's death. Death is a phenomenon that cannot be described solely in medical-biological terms. Death is a condition of life or, if you like, an existential reality. The state of death arises when biological, psychological and social factors combine in such a way—specific for each individual—that the person's life ceases. The medical and nursing professions are most familiar with the biological aspect. There is usually little difficulty in determining when death has occurred, though, as research and discussions in recent years have shown, even this is admittedly less certain than it used to be. Dying is characterized by psychological and social circumstances which are such that the patient, doctor or relatives (that is, one or several of them) knows or senses, consciously or unconsciously, that instead of a particular disease it is now a question of a person who is dying. Dying has many guises, particularly in its duration. A bullet through the temple may make dying very brief and impossible to catch. After a heart attack, dying may take an hour or some days. Dying in cancer may take longer, while in the case of a healthy person after an automobile accident, dying may be extremely drawn out.

While the psychosocial aspect of dying has been neglected for a long time by the medical profession, in favor of assessing the somatic picture, contemporary thanatology is emphasizing it more and more. Attempts have been made to identify psychosocial signs of initiation of dying and to map (Weisman & Kastenbaum, 1968; Isaacs et al., 1971) and describe a transitional—preterminal—stage between a healthy state or some degree of illness and a state of dying.

One needs to have good psychological contact with a person to detect when he or she is dying, as well as an ability to read and interpret the symptoms, changes and signals along the psychosocial course. There are many ways in which a patient may convey his awareness that he is dying. He may wish and be able to express his fears in words but he may also be partly unconscious of this, at the same time as his voice and features, his eyes and his mood reveal his internal perception of approaching death. The picture may be colored, moreover, by the presence of somatic symptoms.

Thus, the chief requirement for assessing the present method's first prerequisite—the patient's terminality—is an ability to detect the psychological pattern during the course of a disease.

General Condition

Dying patients vary greatly in terms of their general condition, judged from psychological as well as physical signs. For the present type of terminal care, the patient must be capable, during parts of the day at least, of talking about personal matters that concern him. It must be possible to relieve pain, difficulty in breathing and other complaints. Severe pain may completely preoccupy a patient, leaving no place or strength for anyone or anything else. For cancer patients, dying may be a relatively long process during which this capability is often present or obtainable with various forms of treatment.

A very poor general status may render the present method meaningless, so that even proposing it may be taken as an intrusion or a burden. It is, therefore, essential that the patient's condition be carefully assessed before the method is offered. This is not to say that terminally ill patients with a poor general status do not need some other form of psychological terminal care.

In my working situation I may, for instance, establish a

contact without any rules or special contract, seeing the patient regularly as need may be. Comfort and reassurance may be the central purpose and administration of drugs may play an important role. I may see patient and relatives separately or together. In some cases, I may ask one of my assistants, a nurse or a social worker to take on the patient. If necessary, I can act as a supervisor.

Intelligence

The friendship relation I aim at presupposes that the patient has a certain level of intelligence. There are persons whose capacity for abstraction or ability to verbalize is not sufficient to make this form of communication meaningful. One should be careful, however, not to jump to hasty conclusions. It is all too easy to underestimate a person whose education or frame of reference is different from one's own, particularly if the patient is full of anxiety, depressed or perhaps plagued by the symptoms of a severe disease. With the terminally ill who have been referred to me, insufficiency of intelligence has seldom been a reason for refraining from an intensive contact.

It has occasionally been necessary to take pains to find an appropriate level on which to talk and a language that makes proper psychological communication possible with a patient whose intellectual resources are limited. The patients in question have reacted favorably to this, interpreting it as a deliberate effort to "get through," while I, too, have found it meaningful and satisfactory.

An example of this, which etched itself into my memory, was the relationship with patient C. He had hardly any schooling and in any event no higher education apart from what he gleaned from drug addicts and prison life. This left its mark on his language. In the terminal course we established a frank, confiding relationship during which we developed a kind of language of our own.

Ego Strength

The term ego strength is used here in the psychodynamic sense and covers the ability to both carry a psychological burden and tolerate anxiety. Occasionally, one encounters a patient with whom this type of contact cannot be established because his pre-morbid ego strength is inadequate or is broken down by the anxiety which overwhelms him when he understands that he is dying. For instance, the dose of sedatives needed to overcome the anxiety may be so large that the patient has difficulty in contributing to a meaningful conversation, in which case the method is hardly suitable.

But these patients are in great need of psychological support to improve their ego strength, as their world is completely dominated by the inevitability of death. One can try to help them by breaking down their overpowering anxiety into components that are more tolerable and then gradually deal with these together. It is also important to select the right sedative or a suitable combination of anti-anxiety and pain-killing agents.

Ability to Communicate

People obviously vary in their ability to reveal themselves to and discuss essential problems with other persons. For different reasons, some people have great difficulty in talking frankly after a relatively short acquaintance with a professional person. The reason may lie in mental disturbances, meager intellectual and emotional equipment, shyness, or simply not being used to talking freely with others. And even moderate anxiety may obstruct communication.

The ability to communicate is assessed by observing the

patient's relationships with relatives and staff, as well as how quickly and in what way contact is established with the therapist.

Motivation

The patient's motivation is of fundamental importance, as the method should only be used if it is clear that the patient feels he needs such a contact. It follows that the patient must realize the true nature of the contact and what it will involve for him personally. One must devote all the time and trouble required to convey this. In most cases, there is little difficulty in telling during one or two sessions whether the patient is motivated.

If a patient is unaccustomed to hospital life or, unfortunately, regards a doctor as an authority who should not be offended, he may have difficulty in saying no to a contact that he does not really want. One has to be ready for this and discreetly change the contact, without hurting the patient, to some other form of psychological terminal care.

Finally, of course, there are patients who need terminal care and would benefit from a friendship contract but for whom I am not the right therapist. In this type of relationship it is essential that patient and therapist "suit" each other.

Special Indications

The method is relatively time-consuming and calls for a therapist with training and experience. It may impose a strain on relatives; patients regard it as unusual. For these and other reasons the method should be reserved for special situations. Examples of such situations are deep, complex conflicts between the dying person and those closest to him, behavior by the patient that threatens his own life, an appeal for euthanasia from the patient, a vigorous revolt against fate, or severe, lifelong problems such as social isolation, a handicap, failure at work, or, perhaps most important, psychiatric disorders. Severe traumatic events earlier in life, e.g., time spent in concentration camp, may make a renewed confrontation with dying and death almost intolerable, creating a situation full of problems.

The special indications mentioned above have to do with the patient's experiences, characteristics or behavior. In some cases, however, the special indication comes mainly from reactions by the staff or others (Hicks & Daniels, 1968). The doctor and staff may be so concerned that they appeal for every form of assistance for "their" patient (cf. patient B), while in other cases it may be the patient's behavior that provokes and frustrates the staff.

CONTRAINDICATIONS

In relation to possible contraindications, it is conceivable that the somatic assessment of a patient is in error and he is not in fact dying when terminal care is proposed. One would, however, soon detect this on the psychological level. Long before a change in the disease and its prognosis has been detected, a professional with psychological insight will have perceived that the total situation is not that of a dying person, that there is no terminality. The contact can be postponed, continued or developed in accordance with the patient's reality, notwithstanding the somatic picture or test data.

This applies even in situations where an acute illness, such as coronary infarction, may very soon lead to death in some cases and to health in others. The psychological contact enables one to read the patient's feelings and needs, so that a terminal relationship can be established if the situation so requires.

This kind of contact with a person who is in difficulty is seldom contraindicated, but since the method excludes the relatives, it should be remembered that a contraindication may lie in the ties between patient and relatives. It often takes the form of a poor relationship between the dying person and his family, coupled with the latter's being against my intervention. In such a constellation, the patient often needs to confide in an outsider. Thus, the method is indicated, but the relatives may constitute a contraindication.

Another aspect arises if the patient is a past acquaintance, close friend or relative of mine. The closer I am to the patient, the more difficult my role as therapist. If he is really close, I cannot function in the manner described here—I am not a "new friend," neither can I "give what the relatives cannot give" for the simple reason that I, too, am a relative. It has happened that when persons close to me have become critically ill, they considered it self-evident that I would help them. I also found it natural, but each time it proved to be burdensome and painful. I felt both guilt and grief.

OTHER CONSIDERATIONS

Having weighed indications and contraindications, it is advisable to consider some additional factors before deciding to initiate the contact. These are the patient's relationship with relatives, his philosophic or religious outlook, his mental health in the past and, finally, the therapist's perception of the patient as a person.

As I have mentioned already and will discuss later, the patient's *relationship with relatives* is of central importance for this method and its application. One should find out early on whether there are relatives or friends who can give the patient meaningful emotional support. The pattern of possible ties and relationships in this respect covers a wide spectrum. At one end there are those who have no one to talk to or are at odds with their family, in which case the method should probably be considered. At the other there are patients with firm family ties and an assurance of support from that quarter, so that there is less need of a special psychological contact. In most cases, the situation is more complex and one has to determine which of these factors predominates.

The patient's *philosophy of life* and relation to religion should be ascertained in some suitable way. In certain cases, the patient is perhaps best helped by a representative of his faith. It has happened that after a few talks I have realized that the patient mainly wanted the comfort of religion. Nowadays a person may be embarrassed about making such a request and the therapist should bear this in mind, withdrawing in a tactful manner and, if possible, putting the patient in touch with someone from the same religious community.

In other cases, there may be reason to continue the psychological contact and also arrange for regular meetings between the patient and a chaplain or other spiritual counselor. Personal qualifications are an important consideration here—religious officials vary in their ability and knowledge concerning the process of dying. During my work at Radiumhemmet I have been able to collaborate admirably with the hospital chaplain, each of us referring patients to the other.

The problems connected with religion, however, are not simply a matter of whether or not the patient is a believer (Godin, 1972; Feifel, 1974; Augustine & Kalish, 1975). Most people in Sweden today are ambivalent or unconcerned about religious questions. Apart from the relatively few who are deeply and truly religious and the equally few convinced atheists, most people have vague memories of deriving security from faith but are conscious of having let go of this. Some, therefore, feel that they no longer have a "right" to this comfort.

A cancer patient (no. 15 in Appendix II) who obviously had very little time left was referred to me and we immediately established a good psychological relationship. Something told me that religion was a real force in her life, so I asked at our first meeting whether she was a believer. She confirmed this in a concise, convinced manner. When I offered to put her in touch with the hospital chaplain she answered just as concisely and definitely: "No thanks, I can manage on my own."

A scientist with a senior academic post is one of the patients (no. 27) included in this account. When I met him at the beginning of the terminal phase, he propounded his clearly atheistic philosophy and displayed a need to discuss it with me. Before he died, three months later, he had procured many theological books and met representatives of various faiths, maintaining our contact all the time. Apart from all the other matters we discussed, it fell upon me to convey to him that the problem of life—and hence of death—can certainly be tackled in a theological frame. I listened with interest and sympathy while he described how he benefited from this newly-aroused religious orientation. He needed to know—and was told—that this is not a sign of weakness to be disdained but that, like everyone else, he had a right to die in the way he found fit.

Patient E came from a religious home and when it was found that her disease had progressed, a doctor who believed in God told her that it was time to reconcile herself with her Maker. This filled her with anxiety and left her very shaken. We discussed the significance of these thoughts for her and during our talks she returned to the non-religious outlook which she had arrived at as an adult. She clearly needed to speak critically of this doctor and deride this missionary activity. She was also able to discuss her atheistic belief, which weakened at times as her disease slowly progressed and her condition deteriorated.

As this method for terminal care is exclusively concerned

with the psychological problems of the dying person, it is important to consider his *previous mental health*. The premorbid personality and mental health of dying persons are subjects which are of considerable psychiatric as well as thanatologic interest. Little is known about how reactions to dying vary with the personality of the individual (Wolff, 1966; Hinton, 1975). Discussions and research about terminal care have largely referred to people whose mental state is relatively balanced—or perhaps one should say that those caring for them have been so preoccupied with the fact that they were severely ill and dying that little attention was paid to their pre-morbid personality or any history of psychopathology. The implications of dying and death presumably differ for people with marked psychopathology, compared with those who are well-adapted, but very little attention has been paid to this so far in thanatology and psychiatry.

There are two sides to this problem. One concerns the ideas and attitudes about death which are held by different groups of psychiatric patients—whether they differ in this respect and whether these ideas feature in some way in the pathogenesis of mental diseases. The other question is how persons who are mentally ill experience the process of dying, what it means to them and how one can best assist them. Knowledge here would unquestionably improve both our insight into the nature of dying and our understanding of the dynamics in psychiatric syndromes. Fear of death has, in fact, been the subject of a few studies among various groups of psychiatric patients (young, middle-aged and old; neurotic, psychotic and others). Psychiatric patients have also been compared with groups of mentally healthy persons who were either somatically healthy or ill (Bromberg & Schilder, 1933, 1936; Feifel, 1955, 1959a; Feifel & Heller, 1961; Feifel & Hermann, 1973). It has been argued that death as a phenomenon has significance for certain schizophrenic patients (Searles, 1961; Lifton, 1976). Deeply depressed patients are clearly preoccupied with their death. Many neurotic patients (Meyer, 1973) likewise seem to fear death or to have the problem of death as a dominant causal factor in their neurosis. In anorexia nervosa, the patient's struggle with questions about life and death can be discerned if one has a close, trusting relationship (Saether, 1974). During psychotherapy in cases of hypochondria and anxiety neuroses, I have had the definite impression that the neurosis was bound up with the problem of death. Similar observations have, of course, been made by many others during psychiatric work, but we lack systematic knowledge of how these patients experience dying when they really become terminally ill.

It would be most interesting to pursue another observation concerning patients who have had mental symptoms of various kinds during their life. When they become severely ill and are dying, the importance of these symptoms pales for some of them, whereas for others it becomes greater and may make dying a time of terrible suffering. This brings us back to the significance of dying for the mentally disturbed. After years of experience with terminal care, it seems to me today that in reality the patient's psychopathology may turn out to constitute an important indication for a friendship contract.

Information about a patient's previous mental health is of great value in psychological terminal care. A number of patients I have seen for terminal care have been to psychiatrists earlier for various reasons, some of them right up to the beginning of their terminal phase.

When she was younger, patient D had received psychotherapy for several years. She had had many conflicts during her life, as indicated by the account on p. 72.

When she fell ill and it was clear that the tumor was spreading, I got in touch with her former therapist in order to learn as much as possible about her case history so as to assess her present situation. When I said that she was now fatally ill, the therapist expressed his sympathy, but apart from a vague psychiatric diagnosis he was not prepared to tell me anything about the patient or the psychotherapy.

When severely ill cancer patients were referred to me and I learned that they had been to a psychiatrist, I used to suggest that they should get in touch with him again. I felt that someone who had known the patient well for a time should be the most suitable person to look after him in this new situation. But most of these patients soon came back to me again, deeply disappointed because their psychiatrist had not given them an appointment. It is not uncommon for psychiatrists today to adopt a dismissive attitude toward persons whose psychological and psychiatric problems, which appeared to involve depression, neurosis or abuse of alcohol, turn out instead to be anxiety over a fatal illness.

A patient in this study (patient no. 34) who was neurasthenic had attended a psychiatric clinic for many years and had then seen the same psychiatrist often. Whenever she had needed psychiatric hospital care she had been admitted to the same ward and she always felt well received. This patient had undergone surgery for cancer several years earlier and now had signs of metastases but was still up and about. Nevertheless, because her disease caused her anxiety and made her feel depressed, she wanted, rightly in my opinion, to be admitted to the psychiatric ward where she felt at home. I got in touch with her psychiatrist who, besides refusing an admission point-blank, displayed toward me all the aggressive animosity which he felt for the severely ill and dying.

The final factor I consider before starting a close relationship with a dying person is *my perception of the patient.* Since the method involves establishing a friendship, I need to feel some measure of attraction for the patient and want to get to know him/her better. In principle it is easy to feel sympathy and achieve friendship in a close relationship with a dying person, but obviously there are people whose attitudes and outlook on life are so different from my own that it would be fruitless to even attempt such a contact. Of course, one should then avoid creating a situation where a dying person may be hurt in any way.

Although I cannot recall ever having refrained from this form of terminal care on these grounds, such deliberations presumably must have occurred to me and had some influence. Probably I then persuaded myself at an early stage that some of the other indications were not present. It is, in fact, conceivable that the patient's motivation was weak because the lack of rapport was mutual.

TOTAL ASSESSMENT

None of the indications, prerequisites and conditions discussed in this chapter is hard and fast — except that the patient must be dying. In each case, one must make an overall assessment in connection with the first encounter with the patient. If one then decides to refrain from an intensive psychological contact, further measures must still be taken on behalf of the dying person. In most cases, one can propose or start a conventional psychiatric treatment, perhaps with the emphasis on sedative and analgesic medication, or perhaps involving a few talks to support both the patient and the relatives. In certain cases, a discussion of the patient's situation with the physician in charge may lead to terminal care being taken over by him or someone else in the team.

In conclusion, it can be said that a deliberately patient-centered method for terminal care, with a firm agreement that excludes the relatives, may be indicated and be highly significant for the dying person in certain situations. The crucial points when following this approach must be: to have a sound psychological reason for giving the patient such care; to offer a reasonable solution to the difficulties of relatives; and to attempt ultimately to assess whether the approach really has enhanced the psychological care of the dying person.

Chapter 7

Establishing the Contact

This account of how I initiate this particular form of terminal care assumes a situation where some kind of terminal care is called for at the time of my first meeting with the patient. In some of the 38 cases I had been in touch with the patient before he or she became terminally ill.

Information in Advance

The prospect of meeting someone whom one knows to be seriously ill inevitably sets feelings and thoughts in motion. There is a variety of ways in which I prepare myself. One extreme is to read the case records thoroughly, study all the information in the note of referral and listen to whatever I can learn from the staff. This creates an impression inside me of an emotional state, of moods and attitudes toward the person I am going to meet. All this will perhaps activate my "psychodynamic fantasy." It is then a question of matching this picture with the reality I encounter. The other extreme is to meet the patient with as little advance information as possible. The circumstances which make this approach preferable are difficult to specify. Perhaps a couple of contradictory remarks about the patient, made in passing by the staff, cause me to refrain from obtaining further information. I lay aside the records and note of referral, disregard the information proffered by a helpful nurse and try not to have any preconceptions about the patient. After an unbiased meeting with the patient, it can be fascinating to read the case record, note of referral, etc. My future relationship with the patient has often benefited from this juxtaposition of two impressions and the analysis of whether differences are chiefly due to other people's perception of the patient, to the patient himself, or possibly to my reactions.

Contacting Patients in General

The first meeting with a patient, be it a single consultation or the start of a long psychiatric contact, involves a number of procedures that are routine but nonetheless significant. The first is to *greet* the patient. Apart from being common courtesy, this is of great significance for the patient. The doctor, e.g., psychiatrist, to whom a patient is referred is an important person for him, the object of positive or negative expectations. His person, manner, attitudes and so on will be observed attentively and sensitively by the patient according to his conceptions and frame of reference.

Having greeted the patient, I consider it absolutely essential to *sit down*. The difference between standing and sitting is full of subtle implications. Of course, if the patient is standing or up and about when one meets him, there is no need to sit down just to exchange greetings and, say, arrange an appointment. But if the patient is seated or in bed, the doctor must sit down in order to come on as equal a footing as possible. To stand and talk with a patient from above is to underline his dependence and assert a kind of superiority. To stand when the other person is too ill to do so and has to remain seated or, as is usually the case, lying down is to maintain one's distance and make a point of enjoying a freedom which the patient does not have. To stand is to indicate that one could admittedly take a step forward and come closer, but also that at any moment one could retire, walk to the door and leave the room. The patient, moreover, is acquainted with all this—it is a situation that occurs again and again in every hospital, every day.

There are many other reasons for sitting down so that one's *eyes are on the same level* as the patient's. A very ill person may find it indescribably difficult just to say a few words or a short sentence unless the other person is very near him. A dying person who is going to say something is often anxious and troubled; to pursue his thoughts and find the courage to be frank, he needs to be in the same position as anyone else who is going to talk about emotional matters—a position in which one can register the expression in the other person's eyes and face. Another consequence of standing while talking to a bedridden patient is that one's field of vision is considerably wider than his. One's gaze can travel over the pictures on the walls or out through the window. There is the risk of conveying, consciously or unconsciously, that one finds little of interest in what the patient is saying or that one's thoughts are elsewhere. This is less likely to happen if I sit down by the bed; we then have much the same field of vision and my gaze is drawn towards the patient's eyes, as his gaze is drawn toward mine.

However long or short it may be, one must ensure that a *talk is concluded*. If I am standing up, it is I who decide when the conversation has ended by starting to leave. If one leaves suddenly and unexpectedly, perhaps with signs of impatience and irritation, the patient will be humiliated and wounded, making further contact more difficult. And even if there is no display of negative affects, such a departure is liable to excite the patient's fantasies and make him wonder whether, for instance, he said something unsuitable or was repellent on account of his disease. But if I talk sitting down, to leave the room I must first get up and in order to do that I must round off our meeting in a reasonable manner. I must prepare and explain to the patient why I am leaving. It is natural to conclude the talk with a remark that summarizes what one has arrived at together, and to agree about when to meet again.

In contacts with the terminally ill one must make a conscious effort both to do what is psychologically appropriate and to counteract the aspects of medical care which the patient may find offensive.

Initiating the Contact

The introduction of a contact for psychological terminal care consists of one or, very occasionally, two sessions. Regardless of whether the patient is referred to me just for terminal care, as opposed to being a former contact whose disease has now entered a terminal phase, this session is spent in deciding together with the patient whether and how our contact is to continue.

After our greeting, the talk takes the form of an account by the patient while I listen. In most cases I say nothing at first; occasionally, an inviting movement of my head or hand indicates that I am interested in listening to whatever is troubling or plaguing the patient. What the patient does or does not tell me and the manner in which he or she responds to my invitation to talk are often extremely informative. The less I say and the more the patient can talk about own thoughts and feelings, the better I am able to watch the patient, observe the pattern of movements, see whether the patient is tense, is close to tears or, on the contrary, wishes and needs to impress me with strength, or is trying to manipulate me.

I listen and note whether the patient talks spontaneously and immediately about past experiences that are still or have again become distressing, or whether his anxiety concerns his present situation or the future and what it has in store for himself and his relatives. Another angle from which I try to assess the situation is whether the essential problems for him are intrapsychic, interpersonal (relations to wife, parents, children), or related to the outside world.

As I listen and prompt with logical but everyday questions, it becomes clear how the patient is adapting. Besides enabling me to form an opinion about the patient's personality and way of reacting, this exchange is meaningful for him, too. He has the experience of talking about something that is important for him while someone has the time and interest to listen. Such a conversation, moreover, serves as an example of the open psychological contact which the patient will perhaps be offered by me.

Assessing the Indications

During the initial talk, I try to decide whether the patient's personality, the entire situation and his perception of this are such that an intensive personal contact, confined entirely to ourselves, would be appropriate and whether I am the right therapist for this from the patient's point of view. In my experience, this question, complex though it may seem, does not take long to answer. The more I can avoid leading the conversation and the more open I can be about the patient's way of looking at and experiencing the situation, the sooner I realize what sort of help is needed in his particular terminal phase (ranging from a short, comforting talk and the prescription of a sedative to the type of intensive contact I describe here).

The patient, too, must find my proposal logical. If he does not view such an intensive contact as consistent with what he has related about himself and his situation, there is no point in offering it even if I consider it to be what the patient really needs. This means that we must communicate about the special nature of his situation. It does not mean that the name of a disease has been mentioned or that we have talked about dying and death—simply that we are both aware that the patient is in danger. It is necessary that I convey to him that I sense or understand how he feels and what he is experiencing. What is important is not the diagnosis or progress of the disease but, rather, a verbal or nonverbal dialogue about being afraid, helpless, alone and everything else that is activated within us by the threat of death.

Introducing the Method

Having concluded after the first meeting or meetings that the present method is indicated, I have to tell the patient what it involves. While adapting myself to his personality, somatic illness and manner of facing his situation psychologically, I have to introduce the idea that I want to act as his psychiatrist and make the implications of this comprehensible to him. I say that it is not a matter of comforting talks or drugs to suppress anxiety but a personal psychological contact; I emphasize from the start that this contact will be strictly private. I will be the patient's doctor, psychiatrist or friend and no one else's. I inform him that I will not be in touch, either directly or indirectly, personally or by telephone, with his relatives, friends or acquaintances, with the hospital staff, workmates or anyone else, and I explain at length why I choose this approach.

In most cases, this offer of a personal, private contact has caused the patient to react with a moment's total silence and an expression of surprise or amazement, followed by an understanding and often grateful smile. Some have added comments such as "I hadn't expected that" or "I didn't believe you could get anything like that at a hospital" or "I didn't know that psychiatrists did that sort of thing." Some have also indicated that I supplied a need which they had not been aware of—chiefly the opportunity to talk openly with a therapist about everything without anyone else getting to know.

To conclude the first talk and this introduction, I explain to the patient that, in order to carry out my intention and keep my word, I shall have to talk with the person or persons who are closest to him—the key figures in his life. To mark the open nature of our contact I ask the patient himself to request the person or persons with whom I am to talk to get in touch with me as soon as possible. The patient should remember that it was he who arranged for his son, his wife or his mother to phone me for an appointment. Having agreed on this, we arrange that I shall return to the patient or that he, if not hospitalized, will come to me when I have talked with his relatives.

CONTACT WITH RELATIVES

The cancer patients at Radiumhemmet who contact me, as a psychiatrist, for problems or disturbances connected with their disease, comparatively seldom bring a relative along to our consultation or ask me to get in touch with one.

The quality of a family relationship obviously plays a part in the individual case but so, presumably, does the stage of the disease. If it is advanced and the patient feels seriously threatened, he tends to be more inclined at an early stage to want to be accompanied by a close relative or friend.

Relatives of the Terminally Ill in General

The relationships between a terminal patient and the relatives are important and have many nuances, favorable as well as unfavorable. When relatives realize or are told that a member of the family has an advanced cancer and that death is not far off, they face a concrete situation which imposes a strain and calls for action. When a terminally ill patient is referred to me, relatives often try to get in touch with me. Sometimes they are anxious to have a talk with me before I meet the patient, and I am usually asked not to tell the patient that we have talked. These confrontations are often charged with anxiety, grief or aggressiveness, illuminating the family constellation and the frustrating, anxiety-provoking situation.

It is not always easy to know how these initiatives from relatives should be met. Therefore, I usually try to see the patient at least briefly before any relatives can get in touch with me. A short introductory meeting with the patient enables me to form my own opinion about his or her condition and our chances of communicating. In this way I am able to tell the troubled relatives that I have already met the patient and that nothing momentous has been said or done.

In many cases, the relatives have been out to give me more or less explicit instructions about what the patient may—or, rather, definitely may not—be told about his diagnosis and prognosis. As a psychiatrist at a cancer hospital, where the problem of communicating a diagnosis is a constant dilemma, I could never claim to know for certain how to act when faced with a terminal patient with whom I intended to establish a close psychological relationship. Consequently, I am bound to tell the relatives that I cannot make any definite statements. I naturally promise to consider what they have said and assure them that my task is not to frighten the patient or increase his anxiety. But what I say and how I say it must remain a matter between the patient and me. If they are under the delusion that psychiatrists are brought in just because something frightening or threatening has to be said, I try to put their minds at rest. I usually point out, moreover, that I have no hard and fast rules about "telling the truth." In my opinion, such fundamental human matters are far too important to be governed by rigid principles (see pp. 25 and 146).

As a rule, the relatives understand my attitude and accept my approach. Occasionally, I illustrate the impossibility of following rigid principles by asking relatives how they think I should reply to a direct question from the patient about whether he or she is dying. This has made some relatives highly uncertain, causing them to suggest that I decide myself. Others—frequently those who have insisted that I do not talk with the patient about his or her real situation—have suddenly said that that puts the problem in a completely different light and that of course I must "tell the truth."

In relation to the relatives of a dying patient, it is important for me to act in such a way that the possibility to apply the patient-centered approach is not endangered.

The Session with Relatives

When I plan to introduce a friendship contract, I get in touch—through the patient—with the relatives for one lengthy and thorough talk. This meeting means a great deal to the relatives. Therefore, it calls for good preparation, has to be held in peace and quiet, and should be carefully suited to the particular situation.

It is not uncommon for more than one relative to come to the meeting. This may indicate that the one whom the patient asked to come is apprehensive about our talk and understandably wants some support. It may also be a comfort to listen together to what is going to be said and to be able to discuss it together afterwards.

Let the relatives talk. The relative or relatives who come for the talk naturally find the situation difficult and a strain. Of course, I know little at that point about their conflicting affects over what I am going to talk about, or the depth of their fear, feelings of guilt and aggressiveness. What I do know or sense about them has been suggested and conveyed by the patient and, although such opinions are important, they amount to only part of the picture.

Before meeting me, the relatives have almost certainly more or less consciously prepared questions, requests or a "defense." Some of them have thought over, memorized and rehearsed what they want to say. Partly for this reason, I nearly always —as with the patient—allow the relatives to talk first. For some an encouraging gesture is sufficient; I ask others what they have been thinking about or I mention a specific event, a form of treatment or an examination to start them talking. But I do not pursue a discussion of the patient's disease, using this introduction instead as a means of getting the relatives to elaborate on their own thoughts, ideas and feelings. This must be allowed to take time. I listen sympathetically and attentively to what they find important in the situation, which also gives me valuable insight into the dynamics in the family.

After a while, we all start to form what has been said into a general picture. The relatives nearly always know—from the patient or the doctors—that the situation is serious and it is essential to speak frankly with them about the fact that the patient is dying. It would be quite out of the question, both in view of the actual situation and on account of the contact I am planning with the dying person, to conceal or gloss over this reality. Together with the relatives, I therefore deliberately try to formulate what we are facing as openly, unambiguously and clearly as possible. How and by whom this realization is expressed depends on the relatives and their way of coping with the situation. But during this talk we must establish between us that the patient is expected to die within a limited time.

Information about the method. The shared awareness that the patient is going to die concludes the first part of my talk with the relatives. I then try to explain in what way I may be able to help and support the dying person. I give a detailed description—tuned to the personalities of the relatives, their perceptiveness and attitudes to the health service—of the method I intend to employ and my aims with this approach. I explain that the chief reason for ruling out all future contact with them is that the patient must feel I am exclusively "his" doctor. I try to make clear that my approach is not aimed against them; on the contrary, my participation may make their situation somewhat easier, too.

Perhaps I say something about the dying person's having many things on his mind that he cannot or does not wish to talk about with them, just because they are his relatives. He may feel ashamed about showing them that he is weak and anxious, perhaps he is afraid to discuss events in the family where he was in the wrong, or maybe he wishes to spare those closest to him from grief and self-reproach. There is no need for psychiatric terminology to explain to most people that all interpersonal relationships are ambivalent and that this aspect is accentuated when one is dying. Similarly, most people appreciate that the presence of an outsider can ease the tensions and serve an important purpose for the dying person.

Much of what the relatives have said during the first part of our talk, as well as aspects of the patient's situation that we have discussed together, are now used to exemplify and explain the ideas in my approach and how it can be carried out in practice. I emphasize that I wish relatives to maintain their relationship with the patient and carry on as they would have done had I never entered the scene. Under no circumstances are my talks with the patient to prevent them from visiting him in the future as much as they and he want to and can.

I emphasize to the relatives that I am a psychiatrist and will not handle the patient's nursing or the treatment of his disease. For such matters they should turn to the ward nurse or the doctor in charge. The practical consequences of my breaking off all contact with the relatives are illustrated in detail. I shall not be available for a talk of any type. Should a relative manage to reach me by phone or should we meet, however briefly, I shall invariably inform the patient about this and about everything that may have been said. This part of our talk ends when I feel sure that the relatives have understood my approach.

The agreement. The last part of the talk is devoted to reaching an agreement with the relatives concerning their cooperation. I explain to them that before deciding anything further I very much hope that—in view of the burden it may undoubtedly impose on them—they will agree to my maintaining this type of contact with the patient up to the end. Here I am more concerned with whether the relatives really have understood and had time to appreciate what my approach means for them than with whether they are willing to accept it. It would be difficult to decline what I am offering—help for a dying person—but if they assent without having understood or thought about their side of it, their behavior later can be painful and a burden for the patient.

In practice, my offer has not been opposed by any of the relatives to whom it has been presented. In most cases, I have not only received their assent but also their loyal cooperation in keeping our agreement.

> The parents of patient A came to our meeting with considerable apprehension. We talked for a couple of hours and they were really able to speak about their grief and despair; meanwhile I made observations about their mutual relationship and ways of reacting that proved extremely valuable during my subsequent contact with their son. At the end of our talk they fully realized what my offer amounted to and what it involved for them and they declared that they were prepared to keep their side of the bargain.

If this meeting can be conducted as outlined here, it seldom happens that a relative, after the contact between the patient and myself has been established, breaks our agreement in a stressful situation. And when it does happen, it is easy to discourage further calls by referring to our agreement.

> Some weeks after our talk, the father of patient A phoned me, distressed and angry after a clash with the hospital staff. When I reminded him about our agreement, he replied very credibly that he had not believed I meant it so literally. When he then heard that I intended to tell the sick boy that his father had phoned, he said he understood I had meant what I said and ended the conversation.

It must be emphasized that *excluding relatives is not an end in itself*. Situations arise where it may be justified from the dying person's viewpoint to make an exception and bring a relative into the talks at some stage.

> A gentle, friendly woman of 50 (patient no. 30), admitted with an advanced cancer, indicated clearly and unambiguously one day that she wanted to be given a fatal injection. This upset her family as well as the staff. I met the patient, we got to know each other and agreed to adopt my approach. She told me a great deal about herself and her life; her wish for euthanasia was never mentioned again. Towards the end of the three or four weeks she had left, it became clear that the patient would benefit if her husband took part in at least one of our talks. Their relationship had always been frank and trusting and all three of us had the impression that the joint meeting which we then held meant a great deal to the patient.

A great deal happens while a person is dying; relationships may change, new needs arise and occasionally a poor relationship may turn into a better one. A joint meeting may serve to confirm this and be of value for the dying person as well as for the relatives.

In some cases, I have introduced this form of terminal care *without talking with any relative*. Occasionally, this was because the patient did not have any relative with whom it would have been reasonable to discuss the matter. In these cases it was, in fact, the patient's solitude which was an indication for the friendship contract.

The situation is different—and more complex for me as a therapist—when the patient right from the start does not want me to have any contact at all with his relatives. The reason given may be that the patient and, for instance, his wife (husband) or parents have such an open, trusting relationship that he considers it unnecessary for me to talk with them. The patient may be right and things may go well at first but difficulties sometimes arise later in the terminal course. Psychological fluctuations in relationships or new symptoms from the patient can result in considerable changes during this final period, which is very difficult for many people. Provided there is a relative who is reasonably close to the patient, I therefore make it a condition that we should meet once before I start working with the patient. An example of a departure from this is the following.

> My contact with patient E, who received radiation therapy and check-ups at Radiumhemmet for cancer of the breast, had been established a long time before she became terminally ill. When we first met, she had given me a credible description of her domestic situation, including a warm relationship with her husband and family, but had also made it clear that she did not at all want me to meet her relatives. When her disease progressed and the question of terminal care came up, I considered that my contact with her could continue and that her relatives would continue to accept their exclusion. If they had gotten in touch with me—which they never did—I would have been obliged to reject them and explain that, as the patient's doctor, I could not be in contact with anyone else.

I would then have had to talk with the patient, explain the situation and ask her—at this late stage—to arrange a meeting with her relatives concerning my principles and my approach. Even if this situation was handled in this frank manner, this would presumably have created some tension in my relationship with the patient.

In some cases I have departed from the principle that it is the patient who should get in touch with and arrange my meeting with the relatives, but I have never gotten in touch with them behind the patient's back.

Once I was summoned hastily to a woman (patient no. 15) with an advanced form of cancer. Her husband had spent the last few nights in her room and when I met the patient for the first time he had just gone home to take a shower and rest a little. Both the patient and I knew that she had little time left and in a quiet but moving way she conveyed her conviction that her husband would agree to any measure that she experienced as a help. Under these circumstances and with her permission, it was I who immediately got in touch with her husband.

In a single case my intended contact with relatives did not come about for various reasons and this, in fact, resulted, regrettably enough, in complications and a strained atmosphere between the relatives and me.

The patient, a woman of just over 40 with an advanced malignant disease (patient no. 13), was married and had children; as far as I could tell, there were strong ties on both sides of the family.

I became involved in her case without a written referral. As the patient had severe physical as well as psychological complaints, the hospital chaplain had been asked to take her on and provide support. Very late in her terminal course I was then contacted by the chaplain, as well as by a colleague at Radiumhemmet who had been a close friend of the patient for many years and knew the whole family. The chaplain, who was due to leave on a journey, considered that the patient was in acute need of psychiatric assistance.

The doctor who was the patient's friend also insisted that I should devote myself to her as soon as possible. I replied that before doing so I needed to meet her husband as well as other relatives, as I had learned that several were actively engaged in her care. My colleague asked me not to wait until I had talked with her husband. He promised to call on him at home that very day and tell him about my work and my special approach to care of the dying.

I then agreed to call on the patient the same day. She was clearly in need of psychiatric support and as soon as she understood that I was prepared to listen, she related a great many things that were full of conflicts and anxiety-provoking for a dying person. Having learned from my colleague that the husband and family understood and agreed to my line of approach, I therefore concentrated entirely on helping the patient and letting her unburden herself of many different feelings.

It became clear, however, that various members of the family had not received sufficient information, had not understood, or in their difficult situation could not bring themselves to understand how I worked. On several occasions during the few days that remained, various relatives got in touch with me for questions, recommendations and other opinions that I was not in a position—after my first talk with the patient—to take up, discuss or answer. I could only try to reply in a reserved, evasive way and this was clearly misunderstood and gave rise to bad feelings.

I realized that this family was displeased with my participation in connection with the patient's death and this is understandable considering the difficulties they faced. But the situation was problematical for me, too. Before contacting the patient I had neglected to have a quiet, exhaustive talk with the relatives about the principles for my method and to give them the opportunity to take up some of their own problems. Notwithstanding the urgency of the case—the patient died after six days—such a talk would have avoided many misunderstandings and solved problems that may still plague the relatives. It is also conceivable that I would have considered the family relationships to be such that my participation with the present method was contraindicated by the family constellation.

After this experience, regardless of how little time there has been or how cooperative and concerned for the patient the relatives have appeared, I have never initiated an exclusive psychological contact with a dying person without first obtaining the approval and understanding of the relatives.

The Relatives' Need of Support

The pain and suffering of the relatives may, of course, be considerable and one can ask who is in greatest difficulty—the dying person or those closest to him. In a book that attracted widespread attention, Toynbee (1968) argued very emotionally that it is clearly more difficult for the latter. He considered it reprehensibly egoistic of himself to secretly hope to die first and considered that in hoping this he was really failing his wife. His line of thought centers on the idea of death as always being a dyadic event. This is undoubtedly true, but I do not see how one can compare different kinds of pain and grief. Interpersonal relationships differ and so do the impacts of death and grief. Without grading anyone's suffering, however, it is clear that the relatives are having a difficult time when I meet them, i.e. when their relative's life has entered the terminal phase. The grief which both the dying person and relatives feel on the eve of death has been termed "anticipatory grief" in thanatological works (see p. 239).

The anxiety and grief of the relatives are not actually altered by the use of my method, but as the patient's problems are gone over in a close psychological contact, a balance may be upset, imposing a burden on the relatives. My exclusive contact with the dying person probably renders their situation more difficult in some ways and easier in others. In many cases the relatives have taken up their own psychological problems during our meeting, in which case I have suggested and often arranged an appointment with another psychiatrist. At the same time, I have pointed out that I will not discuss them with this colleague in the future. This I do lest they should believe that they can influence me through this psychiatrist or glean information about what I know and consider about the dying person, but also so that they shall feel free to express their feelings about me to my colleague.

Chapter 8

Course of the Contact

For the sake of clarity this description of my contact with the patient in the terminal stage has been subdivided into three parts: introductory, middle and final. This has been done so as to describe the course of events between patient and thanatologist in sequence.

INTRODUCTORY PHASE

It is important to see the patient again fairly soon after the meeting with relatives. This renewed contact, like all communication with dying persons, must be adapted to the patient's condition. If there are any particular problems—violent pains, a conflict with the staff or the sudden need for surgical intervention—the patient must be allowed to bring these up at once. Otherwise I am concerned to learn what the patient feels and thinks about the special relationship I have proposed. I want to hear how he views it, now that he has had time to think about it and has also met his relatives and noted their reactions. I need to know whether he is more resolved than ever and perhaps impatient to get started, or whether he is now more doubtful, uncertain or has even changed his mind. Perhaps the relatives seem to be against it or, alternatively, are so relieved that the patient already senses that their visits will drop off and so will their relationship.

123

Talking About Relatives

The patient presumably wonders how I got on with his relatives and their reactions and I have to be extremely careful how I convey my impressions. The patient may well want me to speak respectfully about his aged, somewhat confused yet demanding mother, even though he himself is consistently condescending and scornful about her. He may need to feel that I realize that his mother is more sorry for herself than for him, or that his 19-year-old son is a wasteful good-for-nothing, or that his wife should devote more time to him and take what he says about pain more seriously. He wants me to side with his perception of these key persons while still understanding and respecting their difficulties and problems. The patient subconsciously assesses and judges the therapist both from the latter's ability to understand him and from the way in which he deals with and respects the relatives.

The patient must have an opportunity to tell me what the relatives said after they called on me, whether they are going to keep their—unquestionably difficult—side of the bargain, whether they have been hurt in the final analysis and feel that the patient does not need anyone else when he has them, or finally, whether they defend themselves by explaining to the patient that psychiatry is just nonsense.

Relations with the Staff

Most patients are somewhat skeptical and anxious in their contacts with the various members of a hospital team. Their ambivalence arises because they want to like and be liked by the staff but also feel dependent on them. The staff know things that are significant for the patient, such as the diagnosis, implications of an examination, expected side-effects of drugs or radiation therapy, significance of current symptoms and, finally, perhaps the prognosis. The patient may fear that the staff will disclose something that he is anxious not to know. At the same time, he may be displeased and disappointed that the staff are not prepared or do not dare to discuss all the things that fill his thoughts.

At the beginning of our contact, I make it quite clear to the patient that my promise not to divulge anything to relatives also applies to the staff. I explain that if I have to talk with doctors, social workers, nurses or others to arrange something concerning the patient, I shall always inform him of what I intend to say, to whom and why. This rules out the possibility that one of the staff—by mistake, out of consideration or because of ill-will—will relate something which I have said, done or prescribed without the patient's already having heard about it from me. I also make a deliberate attempt to keep such situations to a minimum.

Control of pain is, for instance, a subject that I may have to discuss to some extent with the ward staff. This form of care is generally handled by the doctors in charge as part of the medical treatment. For patients who are severely ill in cancer, however, the control of pain may be a complex problem, partly because the pain may be intensive and very difficult to treat and partly because pain always has a psychological as well as a somatic component. To this must be added the uncertain, dismissive attitude of the medical profession to narcotic analgesics.

The way in which drug addiction has been handled in public debate, by the mass media, by public health authorities and hospital administrators has contributed to a deplorable confusion between drug abuse and the use of narcotics to control pain. It is not sufficiently clear to medical staff that professional treatment of pain with narcotic substances does not result in a dependence of the type and degree associated with drug addiction.

Having studied the treatment of pain in chronic cancer pa-

tients, I willingly handle the control of pain as part of my terminal care. For this, of course, I have to keep in continual
touch with the doctors and nurses and I always tell the patient
right from the start that I shall have to talk with them about
the drugs he is to have and the changes that may be called for
in his medication. I reinforce this from time to time by telling
the patient with whom I have talked, what we have said and
decided, etc.

The control of pain has not featured, however, in more than
a limited number of my special contacts with dying patients.
Some of these patients are in little or no pain, while the pain
of others decreases appreciably as they approach death. In
some cases, moreover, the ward staff handle this aspect satisfactorily both psychologically and pharmacologically right
from the start, so there has been no need for me to take over.

The Agreement

During our first talk or talks, the patient and I must agree
upon our decision to continue and develop the contact I have
suggested. The patient's particular situation may call for some
modification of details, but generally we now decide together
upon the guidelines that have been described earlier. As with
the relatives, I go over practical situations that are likely to
arise and illustrate how I shall act and behave. The purpose
here is to create a foundation for maximum confidence, frankness and security in my relationship with the patient. Finally,
I make something of a point in this introductory talk that the
patient and I have concluded an agreement.

Expectations

During our first few talks, the patient has been able to verbalize only part of his thoughts and feelings about the contact
we are now establishing. As we continue, his expectations will

be apparent from the way in which he brings up situations from his life, his present feelings, and his fantasies, anxieties and fears about what lies ahead.

My offer of a frank relationship is grasped by many as an opportunity to discuss aspects of their life which they have seldom or never mentioned to anyone. Many people harbor unfulfilled wishes and fantasies about being able to say things and relate experiences or hopes. It may, therefore, be an inducement to encounter someone who will listen to what they have wanted in life, but have not been able to relate. My contact is initiated in such a form and way as to diminish the deeply-rooted psychological resistance which people have to talking openly about themselves despite their wish to do so.

Another obstacle to the frankness I wish to achieve has to do with how one experiences hospital care. People's perception of medical personnel does not generally prompt them to reveal their innermost thoughts in an uninhibited way. As I belong to the medical staff, the patient may have some reservations about me in that capacity. Many patients are aware that, being an oncologist as well as a psychiatrist, I am familiar with their disease; at the same time, this makes me a hospital figure, a doctor in a hierarchy.

Consequently, if the desired psychological contact is to be achieved, the patient must have opportunities to test the relationship which I have described and promised.

Testing

It is inevitable and understandable that in this situation the patient has to test and re-test if I really am going to keep my side of the agreement. He needs to find out whether he really is going to be able to tell me frankly how he experiences hospital care, complain about doctors or nurses, express his feelings about illness and death, revolt against fate or God and really tell someone about himself and his life. If he is charged with anxiety or suffering, the patient must be able to frustrate and burden me and still find that I do not break my promise. He also needs to test my assurance that no one else will be told what passes between us. It is only natural that he deliberately or unconsciously constructs situations that put me on trial.

The relationship I offer the patient is in a sense unique, difficult to name, and hard for him to really believe in. We cannot really make any progress until he has built up a sense of security in our relationship and feels that he can rely on me and the approach I represent (see, for instance, patient A).

However, it is also important that I get to know the patient as thoroughly as possible. The way he tests me, the questions he raises, the aspects of interpersonal relationships that arouse his suspicion and the verbal guise in which he clothes his tests—all these help me to become familiar with his personality and understand how he reacts. The time comes when we both feel that our relationship has become firm, a form of security despite the patient's insecure situation; the initial tesing is phased out, though, of course, the patient may suddenly need to test me again later on.

Such a test at a later stage in our relationship, i.e., not as part of our joint effort to get to know each other, has quite different— and more serious—implications. If this happens, I must try hard to discover why. Perhaps someone has said something which made the patient unsure of me, or maybe he is giving expression to anxiety over a sudden change in his disease. If I am able to cope with his accusation or find a good psychological response, so that the patient discovers his suspicions were unfounded, we can then laugh it off together and thereby strengthen our relationship still more.

But if the patient, having learned to trust our relationship, finds that I really have broken the ties which we formed together, this constitutes and is experienced as deceit, with all its implications in this as in any other human relationship. The patient is justifiably hurt and it becomes more difficult for us to communicate. Just because our relationship is so personal and rests on mutual frankness and confidence, it does not take much to wound the patient and make his situation more difficult instead of easier. This is one of the reasons why I am so obstinate and determined in my efforts to adhere consistently to the agreed rules for our contact.

Structure of the Contact

A certain amount of time early in the contact is thus spent in getting to know each other and building up a trusting, durable relationship. The aim of this contact—to share the dying person's experiences—is then pursued on this foundation. The time required to build up this confidence obviously varies. If contact is initiated late in the course of dying, the patient and I are both aware, explicitly or otherwise, that we have no time to lose if we are to reach one another verbally. I must then attempt to get close to the patient without delay and convey a willingness to match our talks to his feelings. A balance has to be struck so that I do not increase the patient's anxiety either by rushing him or by avoiding or postponing the topics that are most vital for him.

In cases where there is still some time at our disposal, I have found it appropriate to give our contacts the superficial form of *traditional psychotherapy*. The patient and I agree about the frequency of my visits, usually one or two a week, I fix a day and time, perhaps also indicating the approximate duration of each session.

Whatever we agree upon should then be followed consistently for a time so that the patient really feels the existence of our agreed contact. A late arrival, a forgotten appointment or change of schedule is always bad for a relationship. It is considered nonchalant and is therefore hurtful,

besides being open to the interpretation that I am demonstrating the patient's dependence on me or am reluctant to
come. Patients who are dying, who perspire, groan or smell,
are prone to draw such conclusions. One should do everything to counteract such feelings of being offensive or at a
disadvantage, and the least one can do is arrive on time for
a talk.

In this type of contact, the firm agreements have a psychodynamic significance that does not apply in conventional
psychotherapy. This is because later on I alter the structure
of the contact with a particular purpose in mind, inserting
extra talks more frequently and calling on the patient more
often as his burden increases. The patient notices this change,
which I do not need to formulate in words and can leave
him to interpret. He does not need to mention that he is
feeling worse, but we both know that the alteration of visits
signifies this and he can take up the matter at once or later
in whatever way he wishes.

Content of the Sessions

As mentioned earlier, the contact aims at a frank, all-
round communication on every plane between the dying person and the therapist. In most cases, the chief instrument
for this is a dialogue, i.e., an exchange in which one of the
two participants in the contact formulates a thought, a question, a wish or something else and the other understands and
responds emotionally and cognitively. He, in turn, says something in a form which the other person likewise understands
with his feelings and intellect, experiences, and reacts to. A
dialogue is in progress as long as both experience that they
are taking part in an exchange of thoughts, that each of
them is contributing to this, and that emotions as well as
thoughts are being exchanged.

To a large extent, it is the patient who chooses the subject matter. If his physical condition permits, however, it is desirable and important, both for him and for me, to go over his earlier life. But this must never descend to stereotypical questions and answers. Instead, the subjects I raise must refer in an understandable and meaningful manner to what has been said earlier, so that the patient feels I am asking out of interest and consideration for him and not to record a "history."

It should be noted that the type of exploration which precedes traditional psychotherapy, i.e., a diagnostic exploration, is irrelevant and may even be harmful in the present type of situation. I certainly want to assess the psychodynamics in the patient's personality and hear about his childhood and adolescence, relations with his parents, workmates and the opposite sex, and a great deal more. But this is not because I intend to direct psychotherapy at some symptom, some pathological conflict, misconception or behavior which others find deviant. My purpose is to understand the patient's view of his past life, his experience of life here and now, and his fantasies, thoughts and emotions about the future, the reason being that he is dying and needs someone to share this with him. Despite certain superficial similarities, this is not the same as current psychiatric-psychotherapeutic activity (see p. 179).

The phenomenon of "unrepression," which has been discussed by Janis (1958), has attracted little attention in present-day psychology. The term denotes a condition where matter which has been more or less suppressed easily rises to the surface of consciousness. The phenomenon is common when a person is threatened, physically weak, affected by pain or worn out. Janis presents a number of feasible psychological explanations. This phenomenon can be observed very clearly in persons who are dying. Faced with this threat, much is verbalized that had previously been forgotten and suppressed.

This is no doubt a help in establishing my special type of relationship. It also explains why problems and conflicts are often easily worked through in a short time in contacts with the dying.

There is something in the contact with a dying person that causes one to listen intensely and sensitively. Everything that happens and is said becomes significant. Several writers have attempted to catch this specific aspect, which, for instance, is conveyed by the well-known book of Kübler-Ross (1969). In Shneidman's (1973) formulation, the aspects of transference and countertransference in work with the dying are unique and differ in an elusive manner from other interpersonal communication. In his anthology (1976), Shneidman tries to catch the difference schematically between the conversation of a dying person with friends and relatives on the one hand and the thanatologist's professional exchange with him on the other. Writing about his conversations with dying persons, Hinton (1967) relates: "Often we came to know each other well—friendship grew fast in these circumstances and sometimes it seemed difficult to believe we met only a few times" (p. 96).

Obviously, the content of the talks ranges very widely. If the disease remains stationary for a period, the patient has plenty of time to bring up what he has done in the past, his emotional relationships, as well as hopes and dreams that have come true or, on the contrary, been dashed to the ground.

Some of a patient's thoughts and feelings are also revealed in spontaneous accounts of how he experiences the hospital, doctors, nurses and so on. Medical care and its organization create an artificial environment so that in a sense one has a "laboratory situation" in which attentive observation discloses the structure of the patient's personality very distinctly. This environment is a severe test of patients with a hysteroid tendency, compulsive-neurotic features, problems of dependence/independence, or a depressive disposition. Besides being easy to detect the patient's difficulties and characteristics, it is now possible—in the light of the current situation—to understand his earlier experiences.

One aim in work with the dying is, for instance, to emphasize the individuality of the patient in every way. I do all I can in word and deed so that the patient can function as much as possible as an individual. Besides trying to understand and share his thoughts, feelings and experiences, this involves helping him to develop and realize his characteristics. Patients may have talents or interests that they have not been able to cultivate before. They may have an aptitude for writing poetry or prose, a need to help others (see patient E), or perhaps a desire to finish a task they find important. Every measure that assures the individuality of the patient can add a positive aspect to dying.

Though different authors have tried to conceptualize their approach, it is not easy to express and describe what we are doing when we work psychologically with a person who is dying. In my work with the patients, I have found it useful to apply a set of dimensions discussed earlier (p. 21). In every situation and during every session, I ask myself consciously or subconsciously *"where is the patient"* along each and every one of these dimensions. The changes along these lines soon become evident and important to me and give me guidance in determining where to go next, what to ask, how to react and how best to assist the patient.

Medication

Drugs are often used in care of the dying (Goldberg et al., 1973; Lipman, 1975). Unlike the case with psychological disturbances, very few systematized, controlled studies have been made of pharmacological treatment of dying persons. Drugs to relieve anxiety, induce sleep and relax the patient must be applied vigorously. In the terminal stage, glucocortico-steroids also are of value (Schell, 1972).

Treatment of pain is the most important part of pharma-cological therapy. Roughly 70 percent of all dying cancer pa-tients experience pain. In these cases the use of opiates is not only unavoidable, but appropriate. If they are indicated, it is important to give them readily without dissuading or re-proving the patient, as this only increases his anxiety. Person-ally, I have found it valuable to follow the approach developed and practiced at St. Christopher's Hospice in London (Saun-ders, 1967, 1976a, 1978; Twycross, 1975, 1976, 1978). The aim is to *prevent pain rather than treat it*. I have a frank dis-cussion with the patient about how much and how frequently he needs to take a certain drug so that his pain will not have returned by the time he gets the next dose of medicine. In this way, one breaks his fear of pain. As the disease progresses, it is usually, though by no means always, necessary to give larger doses and this is done by selecting a more effective drug, in-creasing the size of the individual dose, or shortening the in-terval between doses.

In practice, I have drawn up a schedule for the patient and adjusted this as his condition and needs changed. One must not, however, depart arbitrarily from an agreed schedule; also, the drug should be administered regularly, i.e., even when the patient is asleep. Some nurses at Radiumhemmet have ap-parently brought the giving of a nighttime injection to a fine art, so that the patient is hardly roused. An injection that is accompanied by a friendly, reassuring whisper and a pat on the cheek does not disturb at all and produces an optimum effect.

In the cases in which I have introduced this form of ad-ministering analgesics, my chief concern has been to make the subject of pain control less charged. Pain relief is a central is-sue in care of the dying generally, but it is a peripheral problem when working according to the friendship contract. If the patient is in pain it must be suppressed by the best method and most effective means available. The patient is made to realize, moreover, that this is a clear-cut right, not something he needs to either beg or be grateful for. The hospital staff, however, sometimes accentuate the apprehension connected with this treatment. They speak with affect, reproaching and being condescending to the patient, humiliating him and provoking clashes. This harms my work with the dying person in that what I wish to tone down is exaggerated and associated with unnecessary emotions.

It should be remembered that opiates, which are usually given to suppress pain, also tend to curb anxiety. If sedatives such as phenothiazine derivates are given together with analgesics, the effect on pain is often potentiated. Some studies indicate that levomepromazine is itself something of an analgesic. It has also been claimed that tricyclic antidepressants can have an analgesic effect and they, too, have been used synergistically with varying results.

The use of heroin at St. Christopher's Hospice has been discussed extensively (Twycross, 1978). In my opinion, the advantages of this do not justify the introduction or reintroduction of heroin into medical care. It is regrettable, on the other hand, that the role of alcohol in Swedish society makes it impossible to use this without difficulties as a component in the treatment of a dying person's pain and anxiety.

Terminally ill cancer patients are usually prescribed many different drugs simultaneously and there is a considerable risk of interaction as well as undesirable side-effects. This simultaneous medication on different indications can make it difficult to assess the response, which may be interpreted erroneously as part of the process of dying.

The medical profession is all too prone to regard dying as a stage of disease, with the result that regular medication may be vigorously maintained even though the patient—as a dying person—no longer needs or benefits from many of the drugs.

Registering the Terminal Course

If the disease progresses, perhaps with new symptoms, this immediately affects the psychological contact. When working on a personal plane with dying persons, one should try to follow every phase in the course and be on the alert for any change.

The ways in which the process of dying and particularly changes in its course exert a psychological influence on the dying person and everyone around him have been demonstrated admirably by Glaser and Strauss (1965, 1968), whose work is discussed on page 243. The description of different courses and the implications of differences in their duration and nature are valuable in clinical thanatology.

Right at the beginning of a contact, I must do all I can to catch and register the patient's psychological and physical status and note every change. During our dialogue I observe the course of the process and adapt my approach accordingly. A person who is in close psychological contact with a dying patient can quite frequently detect a change for the better or worse before the doctors and often even the patient are aware of it (Beigler, 1957). If my assessment and hence my reaction in our contact are correct, this will benefit our relationship. I am able to assist the dying person, besides experiencing our contact as meaningful and emotionally rewarding. In contrast, an unexpected deterioration, not to mention an unexpected death, is highly traumatic for all concerned, including the therapist (Levinson, 1972).

Initially and throughout terminal care of the present type, I try to read the patient's psychological "signals" and to formulate and re-formulate according to the dimensions I have in mind what lies ahead and the forms it will take.

MIDDLE PHASE

The time limits of the middle phase of our contact have been chosen rather arbitrarily. In this method it can be said to start when the psychological contact is firmly established and able to withstand strain and change. The extent to which a middle phase can be distinguished obviously has to do with the course as a whole. If dying proceeds rapidly, it will be hardly detectable in the brief transition from the introductory to the final phase.

It usually takes some time to develop a close psychological contact. Up to a point, however, the shorter the time that remains, the more rapidly the required relationship evolves.

> One of the patients (no. 15) was referred to me late in the final stage of her cancer because she had asked for an injection that would end her life. It took half an hour to establish a friendship, conclude the agreement and explain my aim and approach to the patient. Instead of taking up or dismissing the patient's request for euthanasia, we quickly established a frank, intense contact as we both knew that there was very little time to lose. A few hours later that day, having talked with her husband, I called on her again and in less than another half-hour she unreservedly related the central conflict in her life. She concluded by remarking that this was the first time she had had an opportunity to talk undisturbed with an outsider about a matter that had plagued her for many years. Next day she was already confused at times and a few days later she died. During my later visits we said very little, but a smile or a nod from her confirmed our understanding and what we had achieved.

In many of the cases reported here, the middle phase of the contact lasted several weeks and was of great importance psychologically.

The Course

This period of dying is characterized, on the one hand, by progression and spread of the disease, with pains, difficulty in breathing, invalidism and so on, and on the other, by the psychological aspect with anxiety, depression, aggressiveness, the struggle with an awareness of approaching death, a sense of hopelessness, etc. As death approaches, the somatic picture conforms more and more to a general pattern, the visible characteristics being paleness, fatigue and loss of strength. Psychologically, on the other hand, the picture becomes increasingly differentiated, engaging and many-sided. Dying can follow very different courses up to the end. The basic personality of the patient, experiences throughout life and the ties with or isolation from other people all play a part. The confidence the patient derives from philosophy or religion and other sources likewise contributes to the perpetual variation in this process.

Stages. Kübler-Ross (1969), whose work and widely-read book have unquestionably been of far-reaching importance for the "new" thanatology, has divided dying into stages of its psychological aspects, according to how the patient defends himself against or reacts to the threat of approaching death. The stages as she sees them are: denial, anger, bargaining, depression, and acceptance. This system rests on her impressions and she has not presented a proper study in which they are verified. The eagerness and satisfaction with which this division into stages has been adopted in many quarters are remarkable. It is as though this regular sequence in the confusing variety of dying has given many people a sense of security and confidence.

Among workers in theoretical and clinical thanatology, however, there are growing doubts as to whether people really do "die in stages." These stages could not be verified by either Shneidman (1973) or Kastenbaum (1975a), nor could they be confirmed in a review of the literature (Schulz & Aderman, 1974). Weisman has written (1977), "Schematic stages— denial, anger, bargaining, depression, acceptance—are at best approximations, and at worst, obstacles for individualization." It certainly does not appear reasonable to classify dying according to these few, dominant symptoms or defense mechanisms. Defense mechanisms do have their place in psychodynamic theory, when used in a stricter, more limited sense, but they can hardly be made to stand for the characteristic features of anything as complicated and extensive as dying.

Nor is the question of stages in dying merely of theoretical thanatological interest—it also has a bearing on practical clinical work with the dying. Whatever her intentions may have been, the fact remains that the stages of Kübler-Ross have come to be regarded as a checklist for the process of dying. Each stage is expected to follow the one before it in the given sequence. And if a patient clearly deviates from this pattern, one is now liable to hear from the hospital staff that his dying is "wrong." In this scheme, dying ends with acceptance, whereas in reality some accept but many do not. There is also an alarming element of wishful thinking in letting hospital staff and others get the idea that dying persons will always arrive at acceptance.

I have not found any confirmation of these stages in my work and it would be entirely alien to me to meet a dying person with a preconceived idea of how he should tackle this process. My goal is the opposite: to observe how the dying person is meeting his difficult challenge and assist him in as flexible a way as possible.

Structure of the Contact

It is now that even the external form of my contact with the patient becomes increasingly distinguished from conventional psychotherapy. It is generally true to say that the worse the patient becomes, the more frequently the therapist should visit him. The earlier agreements about regular visits at fixed times should be broken by the therapist spontaneously and in time, i.e., before the patient has realized, or at least before he has verbalized, that he needs more frequent visits. Having previously agreed to make regular visits, this alteration is a deliberate psychological measure on my part to mark that a change has occurred. All one's unsolicited measures, actions, statements and so on reveal to the patient that one understands him, senses or recognizes his needs, and wishes to do something to satisfy them.

The first time I pay a patient an extra visit may coincide with a specific event. A painful measure may have to be made, for instance, and I then elect to be present or to arrive shortly afterwards. Or perhaps I have prescribed a new analgesic against a sudden increase in pain and drop in without warning when work is over to hear about its effect, letting the conversation continue for a while in the context of our regular dialogue. The extra visits soon cease to be extra and the patient learns that I will be turning up now and then and that I try to match this with his needs. Such visits need not be long; the essential point is to be prepared in some situations for as long a session as in the beginning (assuming that there was a beginning in that particular contact, when for instance the schedule might have been 45 minutes once a week) and in other situations perhaps to just sit there for a time and say practically nothing. It is not the length of the talks that is crucial but the fact that a meaningful dialogue continues for a time in such a way that the patient feels that he and I are collaborating, working on his situation and, whatever the future has in store, are prepared to face it together.

Breaks

Any therapist engaged in conventional psychotherapy or some other long-term contact with patients, such as the one described here, may be obliged to break off, which is invariably a strain on the relationship. Suspending a contact is always in a sense a breach of faith. In contacts with the dying, the effect may be still more serious. The closer the contact, the more serious the consequences of interrupting it. But the reasons for breaking off are also important. A break may be sudden and unexpected or planned and foreseen for some time.

Unexpected breaks. It goes without saying that whenever a sudden break has to be made, the patient must be informed that the session has to be cancelled. If it is possible, I tell him or her myself, giving an acceptable and full explanation. The patient will inevitably compare my reason with the alternative of visiting him and arrive at my order of priority. If I cannot tell the patient myself, I must ask someone (a nurse, social worker, doctor) to do so for me, giving the reason. At the first opportunity I must then call on the patient, explain why I did not come, and give him a chance to air his feelings about all this.

The reason for interrupting the contact is naturally crucial for the patient's acceptance of it. A scientific meeting or a much-needed rest will often seem poor reasons to the dying person, who may be hurt. An entirely different reaction can be expected if I am prevented by a sudden illness. A sick therapist can trigger many emotional processes in the patient. Fantasies about being punished still further as a dying person by being deprived of the person who wants to help, or the sudden idea that perhaps the therapist can die "instead of" the dying person are just two examples. My experiences during a period of illness may, moreover, provide valuable material for our talks, giving the patient an occasion to work over and express many aspects of "being ill" from a different angle.

The quality of the contact also modifies the influence of an unexpected interruption. By frankly describing one's own feelings about and reasons for needing to go away, it is sometimes possible to get the patient to understand and accept this. The contact may benefit if it is the patient who persuades me not to miss, say, a chance to relax. It may be significant for the patient that it is he who tells me to stay at home another three days to be certain of recovering from a bout of "flu."

Planned breaks. Different problems arise when one can see the interruption coming, e.g., a holiday, a trip to a scientific conference, a leave of absence for research or anything else that is part of hospital work. While it is true that these activities can often be shifted, altered or postponed, in doing so I still reveal my priorities.

The crucial point in such a context is that a patient with whom one is planning a contact that will last some time is carefully informed as early as possible about a future interruption. After some time, he must also be reminded that I shall be away during this or that period. As the psychodynamic content of these contacts is constantly changing, it will be found that when such reminders are given, the planned interruption takes on a new meaning. Having been accepted initially in a calm, matter-of-fact manner, after a week or two the same information may make the patient feel very hurt and complicate the contact in the future.

By the time of the last visit before a holiday or conference trip, the problem may have been thoroughly discussed and utilized constructively; alternatively, the patient may be extremely hurt and refuse to converse on this last occasion. The latter may be a way of demonstrating that the contact is being broken by him, not me, and that he wants to maintain the initiative (see patient A).

Another difficulty may be that, as a therapist for dying patients, having mentioned at the start that I intend to take a fortnight's holiday, I regret this because the patient has become much worse and the contact so important for us both that I do not want to go away. It is not then just a simple matter of telling the patient that I've changed my mind. He may remember my plan and consider that I deserve a holiday, while regretting that I shall be away. But if I now cancel or postpone it, he will inevitably believe that I consider he has very little time left.

"Middle knowledge"—Avery Weisman's term to describe the psychological state between total denial and total acceptance (see p. 236)—makes these situations still more complex. The patient denies the seriousness of the situation to some extent and to that extent accepts it. The position of a patient's middle knowledge on this scale fluctuates and this delicate balance will be affected if the therapist does something such as canceling or undertaking a planned journey. It is important to follow this process carefully and use repeated assessment in an attempt to evaluate the course ahead.

When some therapists who work with the dying have to go away, they drop a line or phone in a message to their patients as a sign that they are thinking of them. Personally, I have never found this necessary or meaningful. On the other hand, during a trip I have occasionally phoned a particular doctor or nurse at reasonable intervals to keep myself informed about the patient's condition. In this way I have been able to complete or break off my period of absence according to the needs of a severely ill person.

As the patient deteriorates and the relationship deepens, it becomes less and less possible to replace one therapist by another. For the dying person, it becomes significant that it is I —and just I—who comes again and again.

> Patient E, for instance, never got in touch with the other psychiatrist with whom I made an agreement on the occasions when I had to go away during our contact, which lasted more than two years. And yet she insisted,

in keeping with her nature, that I always took my holidays and other opportunities for recreation.

Whenever my holiday has coincided with one of these close psychological contacts with a dying patient, I have either taken the holiday some other time or located it so that I was able to visit the dying patient in the hospital at suitable intervals.

Content of the Dialogue

The content of our talks also differs from that in traditional psychotherapy. Each talk with the dying is certainly a step in a continuous dialogue, but I never know in advance what our subject will be on that particular occasion. New situations and new questions are always arising during the course of dying and they have to be scrutinized and discussed while they are in the air. As the patient is certain that our contact is completely confidential, we naturally discuss personal matters. A problem that is usually passed over in the care of dying patients will exemplify this.

Dying persons may have been ill a long time, which inevitably affects their relationships to those nearest to them. An important component of interpersonal relationships and one that can cause the dying person difficulty is *sexuality*. He or she may long to be close to and intimate with the partner; this is seldom feasible in a hospital and in any event their sexual life together cannot continue as before. The dying person may also feel guilty because circumstances, or fatigue as a result of the disease, deprive the partner of sexual companionship (Leiber et al., 1976). The dying person may have feelings of both longing and of guilt and have difficulty in talking about these with the partner. Jealousy and aggression may be aroused, moreover, by thoughts of how the other person may be resolving the difficulty. These feelings can be discussed in the friendship contract with the therapist.

It is not possible here to even hint at the manifold problems, questions, thoughts and conflicts which arise in this phase. Added to this, people differ, each in his own way, and the manner in which one dies depends on the personality and the life one has lived. The dimensions of dying, described earlier (p. 21), are to me a way of structuring and understanding what is going on. Psychological, social, financial and many other practical problems come up (Koenig, 1968). The aim of my work is to let each person live out his life as far as possible until he dies. All that can conceivably be done must be done to assert the patient's *individuality*.

In this phase, when the contact is firmly established and the patient not yet moribund, the phenomenon known in psycho-analytical theory as *transference* is often very distinct. The patient's feelings for his parents in childhood or for key figures later in life color his thoughts and feelings towards me. For some of my patients, I clearly "was" a brother or sister with whom they did not get on, or a long-lost father, a partner who abandoned them or a protective son. When working with a dying person, it is more important to use this transference constructively for the patient than to take it up and discuss it with him.

The basic situation in this phase is that a person who has been severely ill is now dying. Despite the certainty that everyone will die, the patient presumably belongs to the majority of us who do not want this to happen, who deny it or revolt against it. But in his present state he realizes, or is coming to realize, that he is dying and his world is dominated by this increasing certainty. The psychological implications of dying come to the fore, while less and less interest is paid to the outer cause, the disease. He becomes preoccupied instead with who he was, who he is, and what will happen to him—and that is what we mostly talk about.

Patients occasionally want to talk about their *progressive deterioration* but it is generally more important that I am there and share its course. My manner, behavior, expression and tone of voice convey that I know a change is taking place. At the start of our contact, we may have joked and spent some time in idle chat. As the course proceeds, my behavior must match the patient's circumstances. When he becomes still worse, when his appearance changes, his features become distorted or an unpleasant smell surrounds him, I have to be prepared to put up with it.

Great importance is often attached to what one says about the disease and whether one should *"tell the truth."* The patient, however, seldom asks about the diagnosis spontaneously. If he does, one must pay careful attention to the way in which he asks, what he asks about, and how much he wants to know. It is the patient who is dying and he knows this, deep down. If he wants to talk about it, I do so frankly but strive to gauge how much he wants to hear and, of course, I never burden him with truths that he has not asked about. In practice, such matters are relatively easy to handle in a close, trusting relationship.

Most people consider that dying is entirely negative, but the matter is more complicated than that. Psychological *growth and maturity* are also feasible during the course of dying, as described by various writers (Eissler, 1955; Zinker & Fink, 1966; Weisman, 1972). This maturing process seems to depend on, among other things, how imminent death is for the individual and how sudden its threat. It may result in a renewal of relationships with family members and the forming of new friendships. The patient may have time to develop a new way of looking at himself and life's questions as well as a more mature way of meeting the inevitable. He may derive satisfaction from having a therapist at his side with whom these new experiences can be shared and verbalized.

Much of the *content of our talks* belongs to matters which the dying person discusses exclusively with me. Other matters are no doubt discussed both with me and with his nearest relatives, or perhaps with a friend, clergyman or another outsider. There is also undoubtedly a sector of life that the patient discusses solely with his own circle and not with me. This I should bear in mind and ask myself from time to time which problems these are. I should also consider whether it is appropriate that a particular problem remains a matter between the patient and relatives.

The patient may find it very encouraging if the therapist takes up a theme that has not been touched earlier, thereby displaying his interest, insight into the patient's situation and willingness to talk even about matters that the patient believes to be irrelevant or unimportant, or is perhaps ashamed about or reluctant to trouble the therapist with.

The Will to Die

A wish to die may arise while a person is dying, as it may earlier in life. Many people harbor anxiety about death at the same time as they experience a longing to die. The severely ill may have many reasons for not wanting to live. Such a wish in a dying person can become a demand for action, either a summons to others to do something or a decision to act himself.

Request for death. The medical profession today reacts differently to the patient who wishes to be spared a particular treatment so as not to prolong his pain and suffering and to the one who asks for active measures to end his life. These problems are treated as a matter of ethics and as though it were a question of doing what is right or wrong (moral philosophy). We are enormously frustrated by patients who ask us to shorten their life. We feel as though we had been asked to commit a crime (the legal aspect). As far as our medical obligations towards the sick are concerned, however, the ethical principles are self-explanatory and generally accepted. When a request for death arises, what is needed instead is a careful analysis of the patient's entire psychosocial situation in order to arrive at what is best for the patient in the light of his capabilities and circumstances (psychology). There is a growing recognition that when these questions arise in medical care, what matters is the psychosocial situation of the individual patient rather than ethical considerations (Abramson, 1975; Clark & Levy, 1975; Crane, 1975).

When patients have indicated to me that they would like all treatment to cease or that they would like something to be done to shorten their life, I have always informed them that, before cooperating, I must be convinced that this is the only conceivable way out of their present situation. I have then offered them a private psychological contact, so that I can get to know them and we can find a solution together. With the formation of such a contact, no patient has ever referred again to his request for a fatal injection or the like.

> One Friday afternoon a doctor at Radiumhemmet phoned in the middle of my office hours, asking me to come at once to a patient who needed terminal care. As soon as I had finished talking with my current patient, I went up to the ward and was told by the doctor that the matter concerned a woman of 50 (patient no. 30) with advanced ovarian carcinoma, whom everyone on the ward liked and had been concerned about but who now needed immediate psychiatric assistance. I promised to go in to her at once for a short talk and to arrange a time for Monday, as my afternoon was fully booked. To this the doctor replied: "*If* there's going to be a Monday, that is!", implying that the patient was likely to die before then and that I was more concerned about keeping

my weekend free. As I had understood that the patient could hardly be expected to die soon, I went in to talk with her.

She proved to be a gentle, friendly middle-aged woman who regarded me with warm but serious eyes and somewhat ashamedly asked for an injection that would take her away from it all. She wanted to escape her suffering. Her words clearly expressed that she wished us to end her life.

In that instant the door opened and I was asked to come out by the doctor who had summoned me. In the corridor I also found a senior doctor; they both informed me now that in their haste they had forgotten to tell me that the patient wanted euthanasia. Besides finding this frustrating and alarming, the doctors and staff were clearly hurt and disappointed by such a request from a patient in whom they had invested so much care. The staff overlooked the fact that, since the patient obviously wanted an injection, she would certainly ask me, too. Thus, the interruption only conveyed to the patient that everyone was very upset.

During the time left to the patient we established a close personal contact and she was able to talk openly about her life and her situation. She died about a month later without ever referring again to her request for death.

An appeal for a fatal injection is not a wish for euthanasia. People in Sweden today know that no one in the health service will give an injection in order to end someone's life. This appeal is not an attempt to get around someone's ethical principles; it is a cry for help. It is a way of saying, "I find my existence so extremely difficult, my situation so hard to bear, that I would rather die." In his despair, the dying person asks for something that he knows he will not be given. Asking for something unreasonable from the hospital service is also a way of saying that what the dying person really needs is not available, because the hospital service in turn finds it unreasonable to provide.

Suicide. From the works of others (Campbell, 1966; Dorpat et al., 1968; Farberow et al., 1971; Danto, 1972; Ettlinger, 1975; Weisman, 1976b), it appears to be unusual for severely ill cancer patients to attempt or commit suicide. In any event, it is less common than people seem to expect. Presumably, it is not as rare as these works suggest. Some severely ill persons no doubt do shorten their life by ceasing to eat or taking too large a dose of an analgesic without this being discovered for what it is. Quite a few doctors are prepared to provide a prescription even though they realize what it will be used for. In such cases, understandably enough, the cancer is registered as the cause of death.

Even in countries with a high suicide rate, there are only a few cancer patients who, knowing that their prognosis is hopeless, commit suicide. The phenomenon of "vulnerability" (see p. 237) has been studied in suicides, as well as in terminal patients, by Weisman (1976a, b), who considers that suicide among terminal cancer patients is an unusual and deviant way of adapting to the situation. Further studies of the various psychosocial factors that determine vulnerability among cancer patients may teach us to distinguish those who are likely to resort to suicide, thereby also throwing light on dying cancer patients' vulnerability in general.

Death wishes and suicidal thoughts, on the other hand, are common among the severely ill. Roughly one-third of my patients openly expressed such thoughts on some occasion while they were dying. One must be on the alert for signs that suicidal problems are present and convey to the patient that one has read the situation and does not condemn such a way of solving matters. In my opinion, this is the most important form of prevention. As soon as an appropriate opportunity presents itself, one should then take up the question, talk openly about it and with the patient analyze the reasons for the suicidal thoughts. One should try to incorporate this in the general subject of the patient's psychological situation.

When she realized that her cancer would prove fatal, patient D, who had attempted suicide earlier in life, remarked that her previous death wish would now be granted automatically.

Patient E's revolt against the constraints and dependence associated with her disease was expressed through a recurrent, very strong desire for suicide.

Another patient (no. 3) used her disease more or less deliberately to commit suicide. A traumatic childhood followed by an unhappy and degrading adolescence had contributed to deeply-rooted feelings of hopelessness. As a highly intellectual academic she had fought a very isolated struggle against injustice and her own despair. When cancer of the breast appeared, she allowed herself to be convinced by an old encyclopedia that it was nothing to be afraid of and did not seek advice until two years later, by which time the breast had disintegrated, the carcinoma had invaded the skeleton and liver and her weight had been halved. During my management of this patient until her death, it became clear that, although she dreaded dying, in a way she had welcomed cancer and had sought death through it. It seemed logical and consistent to her that the life she had experienced should end with her being broken down and destroyed from within.

FINAL PHASE

The patient's world contracts as he becomes worse. Past experiences and conflicts, as well as the present, are seen in the light of a dwindling future. It is usually thoughts, feelings and questions about this which predominate now. Some patients state this openly; others leave it unsaid.

The Course

Logically, it can be said that one cannot know that the final phase has started. One simply notes retrospectively that at a particular time the patient underwent such a change that the remainder of the contact formed its final phase. The therapist, as well as many patients, know from the start that there will be a final phase. Only someone in close contact with the dying person and able to read his signals can judge when it begins. I maintain that dying is primarily a psychosocial event. Somatically, the process is diffuse and difficult to grasp, so that doctors with a purely somatic training do not find it easy to distinguish the changes that mark its progress.

Some writers have described various constellations of psychological symptoms during dying and interpreted them as signs of different somatic changes (Bleuler et al., 1966; Davies et al., 1973). They can be regarded as descendents of Bonhoeffer (1912), with links to his concept of "acute exogenous reaction-type." The progressive disease may, of course, give cerebral symptoms, which may be both specific from, say, metastases, and unspecific as a consequence of toxic, infectious or circulatory causes. These studies do not seem to yield any psychological knowledge about the course of dying that is of benefit in clinical work with dying patients. In the present type of psychological relationship, patient and therapist often perceive very distinct, step-like changes, the implications of which are clear and must, of course, be acknowledged, verbally or nonverbally.

Structure of the Contact

As death approaches, it becomes increasingly important that I am near the patient. In general, this is far from being the case in hospital care of the dying. I have found for several reasons that *brief but frequent visits* are best.

The patient is often so tired and weak that he can manage only a very brief exchange of thoughts. Nowadays dying patients receive considerable amounts of drugs against pain and anxiety, which accentuates their fatigue and obstructs communication. But is this medication in fact necessary at this stage? There is reason to suppose that many patients, including those who have required substantial doses earlier, can manage with smaller and smaller amounts of medication towards the end. This does not mean, of course, that the dosage should be reduced drastically, thereby risking abstinence symptoms. It does, however, require a firm psychological contact with the patient in order to distinguish between anxiety, calling perhaps for medication, and physical symptoms such as exhaustion and fatigue. Instead, the problem is often resolved by generously increasing the doses of analgesics and anxiolytics in the final phase, which reflects a lack of training in the staff and their agitation and anxiety about reading and interpreting the dying person's reactions.

One reason why the therapist should call frequently but briefly is the patient's need to keep in touch with the family. For the sake of both parties, a large part of his limited strength should be spent on communicating with the relatives who are close to him. If I expropriate too much time, the arrangement behind my relationship is liable to make the relatives feel ousted. At this anxiety-ridden stage, it may seem to the relatives that the therapist is acting as though he knows what the patient needs better than they do, or they may believe that he is more important than they are for the patient. This, of course, is not the case.

Another reason for keeping my visits short is that we may be dealing with difficult, conflict-laden matters. It is tiring to be reminded of difficulties and problems when one lacks the strength, though perhaps not the need, to go on discussing them. As much is now happening to the dying person on the psychological plane, it is also important that I visit him frequently. Even a few hours' absence is sometimes interpreted as indifference or desertion.

Many of my visits are now spent *sitting silently* beside the patient while he sleeps or is half asleep, because my presence calms him. Sometimes I express closeness and warmth by holding his or her hand or stroking the cheek. There are times when a quiet conversation, a proffered glass of water or adjustment of a pillow, a mutual look of understanding or a quick, warm smile are actions of equal significance and rank. They all continue our dialogue.

In the final phase of a contact, it may become necessary for me to *be available* at very short notice, in practice all around the clock. I may then occasionally have to spend a night at Radiumhemmet in order to be on call. This obviously varies with the individual course. Another factor is the presence or lack of close relatives and the nature of their contact with the patient. In practice, I usually arrange for the duty nurse to phone me if the patient expresses a wish to talk with me, wakes up and seems relatively clear after sleeping for some time or if anything else warrants my presence. This does not constitute a breach of my agreement not to talk with anyone else as there is no discussion with the staff about what is passing between me and the patient.

On those occasions when I have telephoned the hospital at night or during the day to ask about a particular patient, the answer has quite often been rather confusing. In the case of dying patients who did not in fact last more than another 24 hours, I have been informed that they are doing well or even excellently. Similarly, extremely pessimistic assessments have been passed on to me about patients whose condition has been stationary and known to me from several visits a day. This clearly reflects a diffuse anxiety about the whole situation on the part of my informants. No training has been provided in the professional registration of a dying patient's condition. Most people find it difficult to judge whether the patient is unchanged or to detect a change and realize what it implies.

In many cases, the patient descends into unconsciousness, ruling out a psychological contact. Even so, I find it important to remain close by because the level of consciousness may vary, with brief periods when one can be of assistance. It is also meaningful for me to *continue the visits* in this phase. Although as a doctor I know what is approaching and although many professionals see what is now happening as monotonous and foreseeable, my relationship with the dying person renders it important for me to follow him closely as he becomes increasingly weak and finally dies.

It is also important to go on visiting an unconscious patient out of *consideration for the relatives*. If the therapist suddenly breaks contact, after having called on the patient several times a day, this is a traumatic experience for them, a sign that one has given up before the end. It is important that relatives who are really close to the patient are not deprived of the opportunity, if they so wish, of being present and participating in his dying and death. There are certain aspects here which have scarcely been discussed in connection with hospital care. To what extent do we permit or enable a man or woman to die in the loved one's arms, so that warmth and nearness are experienced right to the end? There is a desire for this among people (Leiber et al., 1976).

The process of dying may, of course, end suddenly as a result of bleeding, cardiac arrest and the like. Such an abrupt finish affects me and naturally—to a still greater extent—the relatives.

Content of the Relationship

The dialogue we have been having continues during the final phase insofar as the patient has the strength for this. He is now deteriorating physically, but I can still be of use if I register this and convey to him that I have seen and understood, retaining my composure despite my feelings for him. It is most important that he always feels that I am not afraid of him, do not find him offensive and am close by, traveling with him as far as an outsider is able.

The patient's level of consciousness fluctuates, as mentioned earlier, and so does his ability to verbalize matters that have a psychodynamic content. From time to time, however, he will unexpectedly have both the strength and the need to express some aspect of what is happening inside him; if I can catch what is said or hinted at, our verbal dialogue can be resumed for a few seconds. Something that happens in the room, something a nurse drops in to ask about, or the unexpected arrival and equally rapid departure of a relative may give rise to an exchange of thoughts and an emotional understanding.

In this phase I can share the patient's hope or his "conception of his immortality" or, to use another psychoanalytical phrase, "lend him part of my ego-strength." Although I know what lies ahead, I can share in his revolt against fate, his deep despair or his resignation, besides bearing my realization that inside him the wish to die may now be stronger than the will to live. I try to convey that we who are fighting together must adjust to new conditions but that I will still be there and will not fail him or despair. If the patient wishes and is able, we talk realistically and frankly about what is coming. It sometimes happens that the dying patient expresses indirectly, or even directly, that he wishes I could die with him.

The patient and I now know that the end is approaching. He experiences anxiety and I have *guilt feelings*. He is to die while my life continues. Despite all the promises about closeness and participation, I am going to fail him. I should try to hold down my feelings of guilt, but the problem cannot be dismissed. It arises each time I conclude a talk in this phase and leave to take up other contacts and other tasks or for rest and recreation. When parting we can never be certain that there will be a next time and a "see you tomorrow," besides its implicit "perhaps," is liable to become a pretense. I know this and so does the patient. A desire to take a final farewell may arise during a talk, as may an attempt to avoid everything connected with leave-taking. This ambivalence must be resolved if possible or at least discussed at some level. If the contact has lasted some time, it may be possible and meaningful to round it off and say farewell. I can express what the relationship has meant to me or promise to remember the patient.

It sometimes happens in this phase that the patient becomes what is known as psychotic. He has then *regressed* on various planes and for brief periods or longer his reactions to external stimuli are apparently illogical. The term regression is used by Weisman (see p. 236) for a comprehensive phenomenon with several components—biodynamic, sociodynamic and psychodynamic. Of course, these three forms of regression are closely connected and one of them is seldom present in full without the others. Sometimes, for instance, the dying person voices single words or complete sentences that appear meaningless. Just as psychotic speech is considered meaningless, what the dying person says may appear absolutely devoid of content or context. But the more one is in touch with him, the more one can understand what he is trying to express and react adequately to this, thereby continuing to comunicate.

There have been times at a death-bed when I have understood the dying person's "mumbling," while noting only incomprehension and distress among the relatives. Similarly, I was at a loss when I heard patient A, the day before he died, talking with his parents in the native language of his childhood. By that time he had, if the term is to be used, regressed not only in the strictly psychodynamic sense but on all the three levels mentioned above. His entire existence had regressed and the language he used was a symptom of this.

THE MOMENT OF DEATH

The coming of death has different meanings for different people who have been close to the dying person. For relatives, although expected, it is often of enormous significance. Their experience is made up of what actually happens at the time as well as the memories and fantasies which they contribute. For the therapist, the death has been expected but it is always an event charged with emotion. Having had a close relationship with a dying person for weeks or months, one is naturally affected by seeing him die.

I was present at the actual moment of death of one-third of the 38 patients included in this book. In the cases in which I had a choice, I was present in the first place because this was the explicit or implied wish of the dying person. Otherwise, I tried to judge what would be adequate vis-à-vis the relatives. It was out of consideration for them that I deliberately tried to be present just then or felt it would be better if I were not.

If the patient has been unconscious and slowly fading away, I may choose to be present—even though there is no likelihood of contact with the dying person—because of the relatives' anxiety. We have been meeting briefly more and more often in the patient's room and the relatives indicate that it would be comforting if someone who has seen death before could be present. In some cases, they have said right out that they wish that person to be me, seeing how close I have become to the patient recently. They feel that I am almost a relative.

In other cases, I find it natural to withdraw quietly, particularly if the relationship between patient and relatives has been good. Of course, I also take into account the probability of the patient's regaining consciousness sufficiently to register my presence psychologically.

Yet another factor influences my decision. After a short contact with a patient who dies relatively rapidly, so that we had no time to spare while establishing a relationship, it seems natural to be there right to the end. If our contact has lasted a long time, on the other hand, we will have been able to establish a close relationship and then, as a logical step, take farewell of one another. In such instances I have considered it less important to be present when death actually occurs.

AFTER DEATH

The Relatives

When one of my patients dies, problems sometimes arise with the relatives. This often has something to do with what has happened when the patient died, what sort of relationship the relatives had with him and how they really experienced my role. If I have been present at the moment of death, I naturally stay on, try to look after the relatives and convey my sympathy and fellow-feeling. To withdraw in this situation and consider my task complete with the coming of death would not only be discourteous and unnatural but also appear to the relatives to be an aggressive action. They would wonder and search for my motives.

I have to try to help the relatives to accept me and my cooperation as naturally and undramatically as possible, but at the same time I cannot and do not wish to break my agreement with the dead patient any more than I could or would while he was alive. Usually, the scene is dominated by the acute, disturbing experience of death, so that the relatives and I have been able to meet naturally over and talk about this expected yet painful event. Some relatives have expressed their grief spontaneously and perhaps violently. Others have tried instead to comfort me or have shown that they could imagine that I, too, am affected by grief. Some have quickly ended our meeting at the patient's death without revealing affects of any kind towards me.

In the cases where I was not present at the moment of death, the relatives reacted differently. Quite frequently, it was they who phoned me with the news that it was all over now, sometimes adding personal views as expressions of their grief or their appreciation of my help. In other cases I have not heard from them at all, for which there are many conceivable reasons. This may indicate that they are displeased with me and jealous of my role. It may also represent uncertainty about how I would react if they tried to get in touch. Some relatives have undoubtedly thought that the agreement at our first meeting was meant to apply forever and hence that I would not ever want to speak with them again. This, of course, is a misunderstanding. There may still be many questions, important and less important, which the relatives and I can talk about afterwards without violating my agreement with the patient.

It must be realized, however, that when concluding such an agreement one can hardly talk about its implications for the rest of us when the patient is dead. It is a characteristic of death that while one can talk about its prospect, one does not readily discuss what life will be like when the dying person no longer exists. Although we know that death is inevitable and irrevocable, we take care—bound in a magical outlook—not to talk about what things will be like afterwards. That would be to pronounce a death sentence.

Relationships with relatives after the patient's death have also been an intricate problem for me personally. In some cases I have very much wanted to meet the relatives so as to fill out my picture of the dead person and his life, to talk with them about a person whom I, too, miss or mourn, and perhaps to have my relationship with the patient illuminated through them.

The Funeral

When deciding whether or not to attend a patient's funeral, I consider my personal feelings for the deceased and any wishes he may have expressed, but also the relatives— and the latter consideration tends to come first. If I sense that my relationship with the patient has been a burden on the relatives in any way, I choose not to attend the funeral. It is possible that in certain cases I misjudged the feelings of relatives in this respect and my absence may have hurt them.

Considerations of this kind generally guide me after the death of a patient; however, regarding the patients included in this study, I in fact attended the funeral of only three, where another factor apparently influenced me. These three patients were nurse, doctor and social worker and they were also the only ones among the 38 to have this professional connection.

Psychological Autopsy

The patient-centered, psychological method of caring for the dying must to some extent be a burden on the staff who managed the patient. After a patient's death, therefore, I have tried to meet as many as possible of those who were engaged in caring for the patient during the terminal course.

The "psychological autopsy" that features in thanatology has been a source of inspiration and a model for these meetings, though the resemblance is not complete. The term, introduced by Shneidman (Farberow & Shneidman, 1961), stands for a discussion that aims at analyzing and understanding the whole of the psychosocial background behind a death that occurred at a particular institution. All those who have cared for the deceased are assembled for a talk, led by someone with psychological training and with access to all the relevant documents and records. The intention is to crystalize—as far as possible—why and in what way the death in question took place. The psychological autopsy is thus seen as a counterpart to the conventional somatic autopsy. It was developed originally to analyze suicides or deaths associated with more or less definite signs of suicide (Farberow & Shneidman, 1961). A similar approach to deaths in old age introduced in the late '60s (Weisman & Kastenbaum, 1968) is now also used for deaths after somatic diseases (Weisman, 1974). These psychological autopsies have convincingly underlined the circumstances that death is conditioned by psychological, social and somatic events combined in such a way that at a certain point a person ceases to be ill and after dying for some time—seconds, hours, months—dies.

In practice, it is unfortunately difficult to assemble everyone who has been involved in the care of a particular patient. On some occasions I have offered two meetings and thereby divided the team, which is not really desirable. It is clear, however, that some of those concerned never attended such meetings no matter how flexible I tried to be in arranging them. Perhaps they could not bear or did not wish to talk about their experiences.

The primary purpose of the talks of this kind which we have had is to let the staff relate their experiences. Nurses, among others, become attached to the patient, and when the patient dies, they grieve. On occasion the caregiver can experience more grief than the bereaved and thus become a "surrogate griever," as Fulton (1977b) calls it. Vachon (1978) and her co-workers (Vachon et al., 1978) have studied the levels of stress which nurses can experience when they care for dying people.

Each person usually has something to tell, ask about or criticize. They usually speak very frankly and there is an atmosphere of mutual concern and perhaps relief. It is not unusual for a nurse, trainee or someone else to start crying violently and then describe his or her own feelings or difficult matters that the dying person confided. Others obviously stay silent about what they know or have experienced, which may be difficult for the rest of those present.

It is in the nature of things that the staff on a ward go through many intense and disturbing experiences in connection with death; this applies whether or not there is a psychiatrist with a relationship to the dying person. Many members of the staff make a discreet but important contribution to care of the dying and have a right to support, training and guidance; above all, they need to work through their own emotions. We need to talk together about having tended a dying person, each in his own way. All those who have met, cared for and been concerned about the patient can take part and everyone has a contribution to make. It is important that negative as well as positive feelings and experiences are aired. The dying patient had a right to all conceivable consideration and understanding but may well have been trying, demanding or unpleasant. We are prone to feel guilty if we start criticizing a person who has died; consequently, it is beneficial to discuss the matter, compare one's own reactions with those of others and learn for the future. We can talk about the dead person, about grief we feel, and about our helplessness when faced with torments we could not relieve.

Terms such as "pity," "help" and "be kind" often feature in these discussions. I find them alien and in all training in terminal care, including talks of this type with the whole staff, I try to promote the replacement of "kindness" by fellow-feeling and psychological insight.

The personal problems that featured in the patient's and my confidential discussions while he or she was dying never arise during these talks with the staff after the patient's death. There is no prospect or risk of their doing so because my memory of the dying person and what passed between us still exists in a total psychodynamic experience that I do not wish to reveal. The staff may, of course, be both frustrated and irritated because I, as a participant, say nothing about the core of what happened between the patient and me. Therefore, during these sessions I usually reiterate and explain the main points about my approach. While with the staff, I also try to share their and my feelings, reflections and questions about the deceased, his relatives and the total experience which care of the dying has been for us all.

Part III

FEATURES OF THE METHOD

Chapter 9

Demands on the Therapist

To illuminate the patient-centered approach for terminal care from different viewpoints, I will in this part comment upon its place in medical care, as well as its relation to psychotherapy, describe and assess the effects on all concerned and, to begin with, discuss the demands on the therapist who wants to use the method.

Three factors are required whenever somebody communicates with somebody else in a therapeutic setting: (1) knowledge, (2) empathy, and (3) self-awareness. In the following I will apply and reformulate these three demands for those who want to work in accordance with the friendship contract.

KNOWLEDGE

Psychodynamic and Psychotherapeutic Schooling

As the method has been erected to a large degree on psychodynamic ideas and essential aspects of its structure have been borrowed from psychotherapeutic techniques, the therapist should be schooled in these disciplines. Psychoanalytical training may certainly prove valuable but is not a precondition for practicing the method. An appropriate training would seem to include knowledge of psychodynamics, and the skills to use this knowledge, and likewise skills and knowledge of social psychiatry.

The psychodynamic frame of reference in a wide sense is, in my opinion, the only one that is suitable and meaningful to apply to psychological work with the dying. My own experience supports this, as does my reading and discussions with active clinical thanatologists. But in certain respects I also consider that this frame is too narrow. Questions about life and death can hardly be contained satisfactorily in psychodynamic theory, since aspects of anxiety and death-anxiety have been dealt with too one-sidedly there. It is necessary to know something about existentialist thinking and to be willing to see these questions in a wider context. Efforts in this direction have been made by attempting to combine existentialist thought and psychodynamics (Weisman, 1965; Holt, 1975). Lifton (1976) has tried to incorporate death in a comprehensive psychological system.

The therapist also needs to be familiar with social aspects of death, as well as with its cultural and religious sides. Fiction is another invaluable source for extending one's horizons and becoming more sensitive to the nuances of life and death.

Thanatological Knowledge and Experience

Those wishing to practice clinical thanatology need a good grounding in basic thanatology and skills in caring for the dying. Knowledge about death is to be found in a wide range of book on psychiatry, psychology, sociology and anthropology. Some basic surveys are presented on p. 221.

A theoretical foundation is, however, not only inadequate but often definitely unsuitable as the sole basis for work with the dying. Most people have little or no experience of dying persons and find contact with them so burdensome that personal experience is absolutely essential. As discussed elsewhere, the method I describe is only one conceivable approach—and a very special one at that. Those wishing to use it should be well versed in general psychological care of the dying. In other words, they should have worked with dying persons, starting perhaps with the cautious and relatively distant relationship that is common in hospital care. Depending on their interest and aptitude, they should have deepened and improved their contacts with dying persons and should preferably have managed such patients under the guidance of someone who is qualified in terminal care.

EMPATHY

Without empathy one cannot really understand another person. Empathy has to do partly with identification; it is a component of good acting, is essential in spiritual care, and should be present in all psychotherapy. In the patient-doctor relationship, empathy is an important, desirable component. The term has been interpreted somewhat differently by different writers. Katz (1963) has presented a comprehensive discussion. Empathy is an intricate problem in psychoanalytical theory (Greenson, 1960) and it may help to understand this concept if one analyzes the distinction between pity, sympathy and empathy (Wilmer, 1968).

Pity is a composite concept and often includes some measure of empathy. But pity can be a defense against subconscious feelings of ill-will. It can include an element of contempt and is often associated with relationships where one person is healthy (strong, wealthy, large) and the other sick (weak, poor, small). The patient senses this; while noting the pity, he is often wounded by it.

Sympathy implies feeling for someone ("If I were in his place . . ."). It has a positive charge but is aimed at someone as it were from outside. The commonplace hospital phrase, "I know just how it feels, dear," does not help much. The nurse does not know what it feels like to be dying, and even if she did, it would not help, because while the patient is in fact dying, the nurse is not.

Empathy is comprehending another person, feeling one's way into and sharing the other's reality ("if I were him. . ."). It thus involves identification and at the same time a maintained awareness of one's own feelings.

In the process of dying, pity may be harmful, sympathy of little use, whereas empathy is a precondition for really assisting the dying person.

In the present method, which focuses so exclusively on the patient, it is essential to strive consciously and purposefully for maximum empathy. To the best of my ability, through an open relationship that is entirely our own, I try to comprehend who the dying person is and what, in a dialogue on every level, he wishes to convey. I try to identify myself, enter into how it would feel if I were him and in the same situation. At the same time, I try to analyze the feelings which this identification arouses in me. I know in my mind that I am not dying just then, but I also know that my time will come. The anxiety this causes me can be shared with the dying person, together with the means that I use to master this and other feelings generated by the shared experience.

Empathy in this relationship also involves the understanding of the need for continuity and therefore willingness to hold on all the way.

The goal is to strive to get close to someone else's experience, comprehending and sharing it emotionally to the extent that this is possible. The fact that I nevertheless remain outside and "desert" when the time comes is in a way a shortcoming; at the same time, the dying person can experience that someone who is not in danger is willing and able to share the situation.

Flexibility

Just as people's lives take different forms, so do their deaths differ psychologically. The five case histories given (see Chapter 5) are all about dying and still they represent different worlds. One reason why I doubt whether my approach can be labeled psychotherapy, despite the similarities, is perhaps that most psychotherapeutic techniques presuppose that a firm theoretical system is applied consistently in clinical practice. In care of the dying, on the other hand, flexibility is a must and to use a fixed system would be to misconstrue the art. One is not trying to help the patient to function better "afterwards" but to make the limited life he has left as bearable, meaningful and self-fulfilling as possible. This naturally calls for maximal flexibility within a framework of stable continuity.

As already indicated, a dialogue with a dying person covers a great many questions, problems and conflicts in varying guises. Different matters come up in quick succession, sometimes more or less simultaneously, and a particular affect or need may suddenly be replaced by its opposite. To cope with this the therapist must be flexible.

Nearness and Distance

In all personal relationships there is a certain degree of nearness and a corresponding degree of distance. These are complementary aspects, involving a number of components such as empathy and identification. In a patient-doctor relationship, identification is a significant factor. Doctors who are in daily touch with severely ill persons identify themselves with them to varying degrees, consciously or subconsciously. The basis for this identification may be the disease. Some doctors perceive certain diseases (e.g., cancer, cardiac infarction or multiple sclerosis) as particularly threatening, in which case an identification may cause them to avoid a close contact with such patients. Others, on the contrary, choose that particular speciality in order to "overcome" the enemy. The identification may also arise with the patient's person or situation, e.g., nationality, age or occupation in common, or the fact of having gone to the same school.

Some degree of identification is inevitable when tending the severely ill, particularly if the patient is dying—we shall all have to face what he is facing now.

Identification is by no means invariably detrimental. It enables us to enter into another person's situation. But a therapist will be of little use or directly harmful if identification reaches a point where all psychological boundaries between him and the patient dissolve and he is flooded with anxiety, pity and even a revolt against dying. A distance or boundary of some sort must be maintained. It may seem confusing to expect a therapist to achieve identification and distance simultaneously. This is the type of paradox described by Eissler (see p. 225). To the living, death in a sense is a paradox and this has implications for those who tend the dying. This critical situation highlights the paradox of life: having been born, we live and will cease to be.

In the terminal friendship relationships, the fact that I have not known the patient earlier makes it easier to maintain the balance between psychological nearness and distance. Accordingly, it is a greater burden to care for patients whom I have managed for some time before they became terminally ill or whom I have known outside the hospital. Giving this special form of psychological care to relatives or friends is almost more than one can bear.

SELF-AWARENESS

Many psychological factors influence the therapist's ability to care for the dying. The feelings aroused in him by dying persons, his attitudes toward dying and death and his, often subconscious, defense mechanisms all play a part. Some degree of self-knowledge is, therefore, essential in work of this type. It is important to learn to master one's own difficulties, see through weakness and analyze attitudes. Our ability to do all this obviously varies and personal psychotherapy may be indicated. It would be naive to expect "complete" awareness and an insight into the whole structure of one's psychological personality. This may be feasible but is definitely rare. What is important is a will to self-analysis, coupled with assistance when necessary in achieving some degree of self-awareness.

Some areas where self-knowledge is of major importance are the therapist's anxiety-tolerance, his guilt feelings, his need for omnipotence and his tolerance of narcissistic violation.

Anxiety-tolerance

The contact with dying patients inevitably arouses the therapist's own anxiety over illness, suffering, death and the transcience of life. The strain may be very considerable at times and persons with a marked death-anxiety that is easily aroused should refrain from undertaking work of this type. It would, however, be unrealistic to propose that this work should be reserved for therapists with no death-anxiety. It would be wishful thinking to suppose that death-anxiety can be completely eliminated by psychotherapy. Neither does this seem particularly desirable.

Most people entertain some anxiety about death—consciously or unconsciously, at times or continuously—and in order to comprehend the death-anxiety of others one needs at times to be "in touch with" one's own. The criterion is not a certain degree of death-anxiety so much as a certain tolerance of this, i.e., an ability to stand up to personal death-anxiety and that of others, to know and understand what it is about, and to be able to bear it (Feifel et al., 1967).

Guilt

People may fall ill, get hurt in an accident or by someone else, and after dying for a time, their life ends. Suffering often generates feelings of guilt in others, but the therapist who wishes to support dying persons must try as far as possible to rid himself of such feelings. He must work on the tendency, experienced by every doctor and therapist, to feel guilty about what is happening to the patient. This feeling, which may be conscious or subsconscious, is one of the reasons why doctors withdraw from dying patients. A dying patient registers such a guilt feeling and in order to spare the therapist and retain the contact he may conceal his own anxiety and avoid talking openly about his experiences.

Another aspect of guilt feelings concerns the twin roles which the therapist is bound to play. No matter how much one can contribute in a personal relationship, the fact remains that one is going to survive and this generates guilt feelings. In the work described here I have also experienced guilt each time I left a dying person (see p. 156).

It takes a conscious effort to realize and convey to a dying person that one is neither guilty nor responsible for his suffering, pain, anxiety and eventual death. This does not mean that one should withdraw somewhat and no longer engage with the patient. On the contrary, this awareness helps to get as close as possible. Guilt feelings inevitably separate people, while an awareness that no guilt is involved enables them to come closer.

The realization that dying is a general condition, which sooner or later will apply to oneself, motivates support of another person, not out of guilt but from a sense of solidarity.

Omnipotence

A need for omnipotence is present in the medical profession, as in other occupations. It is necessary to be on the alert for this. Owing to the historical and psychological evolution of the doctor's role, it always contains some feeling of omnipotence. The extent to which this is a problem for the individual doctor naturally depends on his personality. An overwhelming need to decide for others is hardly compatible with the care of dying persons. They will be forced to die in accordance with the dominant person's norms and ideas.

Here, too, it is not a question of being entirely free from every need to dominate and direct. The important point is to be conscious of this, constantly question one's own motives and be as candid as possible about working to correct behavior that serves oneself rather than the patient. The closer and more intense the psychological contact, the less must one need to dominate and decide. Otherwise, instead of providing help and relief, one is liable to humiliate and hurt.

Narcissistic Violation

This concept, borrowed from psychoanalytic terminology, stands for the difficulty we experience in accepting a failure in what we regard as a central area for us as an individual or as members of a group. On the psychological plane, the death of a patient is a narcissistic injury for the doctor—a defeat for him in his aims and efforts on behalf of the patient. This is painful for the doctor, but it also involves a risk that he will, say, react with aggressiveness toward the patient.

The present type of work, in which each patient is going to die, involves a recurrent risk of narcissistic violation. Those who practice terminal care should allow for and work on this problem.

Awareness of Motives

Working with dying persons is anxiety-provoking and an essential point is the question of motivation. A clear and deliberated motivation is required of the therapist. What this amounts to is regrettably difficult to specify. There are people who seem motivated and even eager to work with the dying, but the motive, when carefully scrutinized, proves to be a wish to solve personal, sometimes neurotic, problems. Though it is not an easy task to keep those people away from the dying, they are in fact unfit for this kind of work.

As stressed before, the self-awareness of the therapist must be used to scan and be aware of one's own motives.

THE THERAPIST'S NEED FOR SUPPORT

As I see the goals of psychotherapy, a person practicing it in some form must do more than simply talk with the patient in accordance with a particular theory, however sound this may be. In psychotherapy for neurotic and even psychotic disturbances, the therapist is bound to get involved—he has to achieve an open relationship and be prepared to give of himself. In genuine psychotherapy, it is not only the patient but also the therapist who is influenced and altered. This aspect, which many authors have discussed, is particularly burdensome in close psychological relationships with the dying (Shneidman, 1973). The general view, which tallies with my experience, is that one can hardly bear to have concurrent therapeutic relationships with more than a few dying patients.

Therapists in this field obviously can and should have access to supervision in order to go over and clarify their own reactions and conflicts. Such a facility, however, is often limited by the shortage of proficient therapists.

For persons working with dying patients, the chief means of unburdening may be found in their immediate personal surroundings. It is a great asset to have a family with whom one can ventilate feelings. Invaluable support can be derived from members of one's family who convey, verbally or nonverbally, a realization that one may feel fatigue, anxiety and grief and who consider that it is right to do the work one is doing.

Chapter 10

Place of the Method in Medical Care

Admittedly, the method described in this book has its roots in psychology-psychiatry, but I have developed and gradually integrated it in a highly specialized form of oncological care. In order to discuss its place in medical care, the method must, therefore, be seen in relation to physical as well as to psychological-psychiatric care.

IS THIS TREATMENT?

There is reason to consider whether this method for psychologically supporting dying cancer patients, integrated in medical care, is or is not to be regarded as therapy or treatment, terms that are used so frequently and unreflectingly in medical care. For historical reasons, medical care today—with the exception of psychiatry, which I leave to one side for the moment—is dominated by a one-sided biological approach. As a result, treatment refers very largely to the cure of somatic conditions and the psychological aspect of medical care leads a subordinate existence. From this traditional view of medical care, the method described here can perhaps not be looked upon as therapy.

Disease, suffering and death invariably have, however, both

a psychological and a somatic aspect and the contrast between a psychological approach and the traditional biological-technical line is particularly clear in care of the dying. During the process of dying, it is with psychological measures that one can, to some extent, relieve anxiety, agitation, solitude and depression and make life for the dying person somewhat easier to bear. In my view, this is therapy.

Furthermore, our therapeutic thinking is preoccupied with achieving a cure or a definite improvement. Our training and attitudes in medical care have not equipped us to register the nuances of a downward course and a progressive deterioration or to detect what is important and necessary in such a phase. At least we are not accustomed to regard such measures as treatment. Since the patient is dying, we can neither effect a cure nor alter the situation, but it may be possible to relieve many complaints for a time and there is much which can still be done that deserves to be described as therapy.

In addition to all the symptoms of dying that require therapy—somatic but still more psychological—there is still another aspect of death, and hence to a certain extent of dying, which places it outside or beyond disease, therapy and medical care. As has been pointed out repeatedly in this book, death is not a disease. However one puts it—that death is an existential problem, a paradox or a mystery—the fact remains that birth, life and death are more than just biology and psychology. Death's unique significance for us explains why problems during the process of dying cannot only be resolved by "treatment." In our present society, it is the health service that has the great responsibility of handling death. While the medical and psychological quality of terminal care must be as good as possible, it is also essential that people feel that the health service is prepared to meet existential questions. Opinions may differ about whether this is a form of therapy.

IS THIS PSYCHOTHERAPY?

In terms of traditional psychiatry, psychological terminal care is a very special activity. Psychological reactions to somatic disease are beginning to attract attention but psychiatry today is hardly concerned with existential problems. Psychiatric medicine, moreover, is often unacquainted with care of the dying. The method described here is close to psychotherapy, but even in that context it is a special and, it might be said, exclusive field. As we have seen, while this method is related to psychotherapy, the two are not identical.

When discussing this method, many psychotherapists and even psychoanalysts have spontaneously assured me quite emphatically that this type of terminal care is actually psychoanalysis. There is no factual basis for this, however, partly because I am not a psychoanalyst and do not have training in psychoanalysis. This is so even though I have some knowledge of psychoanalytical theory, have had valuable discussions about my method with psychoanalysts and, as mentioned earlier, been supervised by an experienced psychoanalyst.

Some writers who have worked with psychological terminal care refer to their own method as psychotherapy (Rosenthal, 1957; Bard, 1959; LeShan & LeShan, 1961; Cramond, 1970; Stedeford, 1979). A special term has even been proposed: thanatopsychotherapy (Howard, 1961). In most books on psychological care of the dying, however, the question is not considered and no specific label is used. Some of those who at times use the term psychotherapy do so half-heartedly and without any explanation.

Definition. Before going any further it is necessary to clarify what is meant by psychotherapy. There are innumerable definitions, but for this discussion it seems both sufficient and reasonable to refer to a formal definition given by a Swedish group of experts:

Psychotherapy is
a) systematic, aim-directed measures
b) based on psychological theory and method
c) intended to affect the whole personality or such thoughts, feelings, impulses, relationships, psycho-somatic symptoms, etc., as are experienced as troublesome by the individuals or by their surroundings
d) undertaken by persons trained for the purpose who practice psychotherapy as a profession or as part of an appointment for human welfare.

Although they may vary in wording or emphasis, most attempts at a definition are basically rather similar. These definitions, as well as most textbooks that scrutinize and discuss them, assume without comment that apart from the disturbance in question, candidates for psychotherapy will be healthy.

The question of what to do if the patient has a somatic disease is mentioned in the occasional paper or textbook but always briefly and in rather general terms. It is seldom acknowledged that perhaps a somatic disease is causing the psychological disturbance. On the other hand, there are several reports on patients who have become somatically ill or died while undergoing psychotherapy. One learns that the therapeutic technique is altered considerably when the patient starts to die and that the new situation is handled very differently by different psychotherapists (Sandford, 1957; Young, 1960; Joseph, 1962).

In psychotherapy one assumes that the patient is prepared to spend the time, work and any expense that are necessary and accepts the strain imposed by the therapy. It is expected that he will benefit from the therapy, functioning better, more maturely and without certain symptoms, etc.—preferably for a long time to come. Clearly, psychotherapy, in the usual sense, is intended for the physically healthy and in any event not for persons who are dying.

It may be instructive to consider a situation that lies somewhere in between that of, say, a healthy young person who is considered to need psychotherapy for neurotic disturbances and a dying person, i.e., someone for whom there can be no question of a "lasting benefit." What I have in mind is psychotherapy for old people. The resistance to this is considerable, a common argument being that the elderly are too rigid psychologically; others say quite openly that the effort would be wasted because these persons have so little time left (which is by no means certain). Clearly, among therapists themselves there is an emotional resistance; the prospect of sharing what they believe constitutes old age fills them with hopelessness and anxiety (Kastenbaum, 1963).

Goals. In psychological care of dying persons one knows that the patient will die, but wishes to support him in the process of dying. One is aware that for the patient there can be no question of future benefit. It is thus primarily in the goals that psychological terminal care differs from psychotherapy. It seems to me that this difference helps to explain why psychological terminal care is so unusual even in countries where psychotherapy is an established and widespread activity.

Structure. Psychological terminal care, like psychotherapy, is based on psychological theories and methods and to this extent one can say that the two are related. Psychotherapy usually follows a definite routine. The frequency of sessions and their duration are agreed upon at the beginning of therapy and departures from this are considered to have unfavorable implications, the significance of which depends on whether the cause lies with the therapist or the patient. In contacts with dying persons, flexibility, increasingly frequent visits and variations in their duration are both necessary and desirable.

In order to make my point explicit, I will simplify things a bit and refer to "classical" psychotherapy. Here, the therapist tries to assess the patient's psychological equipment, symptoms, conflicts, etc.; he then processes the problem step by step in the light of this insight and his theoretical schooling. Even though the patient may resist, the therapist often has to insist on processing a particular psychological aspect methodically. He tries to follow a plan, knowing what he is aiming at from one talk to the next. When the time comes, he decides to switch to another set of problems.

In a psychological contact with a dying person, it is largely the patient who decides what subjects to take up and what psychological motives to analyze. When a person is dying, the content of the talks varies continuously. The absence of a relative at visiting time, the appearance of a new symptom or the loss of some function—such things arouse anxiety and have to be considered immediately. The patient may suddenly need to return to his solution of a problem as a child, the real nature of the relationship with his wife or the meaning of belonging to a particular community. When he arrives, the therapist seldom knows what will come up. He may be expected to listen to something entirely new, catch on to a theme from an earlier phase, be quick to adjust the talk to a deterioration in the patient since their last meeting, or simply convey trust and fellow-feeling with warmth and empathy.

The structure and course of the dialogue in psychological terminal care are thus essentially different from psychotherapy. It may happen, of course, that a brief period in a terminal contact needs to be spent on a psychotherapeutic exploration or treatment of a limited conflict, unresolved emotional tie or misconception; success here could naturally be a welcome, meaningful incident while the patient is dying.

To judge from the literature (Wahl, 1958; Rosenthal, 1963; Stern, 1968), it is unusual in conventional psychotherapy to consider death, death-anxiety and problems relating to death.

On the other hand, regular psychotherapy with the aim of insight may be contraindicated for dying persons. The diminishing ego-strength and particular situation of dying persons obviously require that they be spared the anxiety that is elicited by all psychotherapy worth the name (Rosenthal, 1957).

Content. Psychotherapy is a large, comprehensive concept. Instead of concentrating on goals and structure, one can consider the content of a psychological approach. The essential qualities in successful psychotherapy have been formulated by Truax and Carkhuff (1967) as accurate empathy, non-possessive warmth and genuineness. This distillation of the psychotherapeutic process reveals a clear similarity between the essence of psychological terminal care as described here and psychotherapy. The extent to which it is reasonable or desirable to characterize this approach as psychotherapy is largely a question of which aspects of psychotherapy one emphasizes and how far one accepts departures from accepted psychotherapeutic "techniques."

There is another side to this question which ought to be mentioned here. There is a tendency to use the term psychotherapy very loosely in medical care. Doctors often say and somatic textbooks state that, in addition to specific treatments for a disease, the patient should also have psychotherapy. I am frequently asked to give the patient "a little" psychotherapy.

Besides belittling psychotherapy, this reveals an ignorance of what it does and does not involve and the variety of forms it can take. For this reason, too, it seems desirable to reserve the term psychotherapy for methods of psychological treatment that are clearly defined and delimited. One can then consider whether it is meaningful and/or desirable to describe this method for psychological care of the dying as psychotherapy. This question has been discussed recently by Feigenberg and Shneidman (1979).

IS THIS CONFESSION?

Something should be said about whether my approach is comparable to confession. Certain components—the exclusion of others, freedom to talk frankly about oneself—may resemble such a situation. But in a confession one talks about conscious events, questions, feelings and so on, whereas the psychological contact with a dying person is just as much concerned with unconscious sources of anxiety, conflicts and experiences.

Confession, moreover, aims at repentance, penitence and forgiveness in a religious setting. In making it easier for the patient to express his personal feelings, my contact does not imply that I do or do not convey forgiveness in a religious sense. I am concerned instead to share with the dying person his experiences during life, including this dying phase. I try to convey that I understand him and hope that together we can see his present condition as a part of life that we shall all go through. I neither condemn nor forgive; I share his experience of human companionship.

APPLICABILITY IN DISEASES OTHER THAN CANCER

As this approach to care of the dying was developed by me at Radiumhemmet, the subjects were patients with cancer. The original disease of a dying patient is, however, of secondary importance. The crucial question with this method is not whether a particular disease is present but whether there are the indications, conditions and time for establishing a psychological relationship.

Besides patients with cancer, for whom dying is often relatively protracted, there are many patients with heart complaints or, for instance, chronic diseases, for whom psychological terminal care of this type could be appropriate. It would obviously not be applicable in acute cardiac infarction, if the patient remains unconscious until he dies, or after severe brain injuries which leave the patient unconscious for a long time. On the other hand, as soon as patients with cardiac infarction become conscious again, they should receive all possible psychological support. When an open contact has been established, it will be clear whether this should develop into psychological terminal care. After an infarction, every patient needs someone with whom to talk properly and many may need psychological terminal care of the type described here. Regardless of whether they die after a time, perhaps not until a re-infarction, or recover, their psychosocial situation is so anxiety-provoking that they require qualified psychological support (Chandler, 1965; Hackett & Weisman, 1969; Hackett & Cassem, 1972; Weisman, 1972, p. 79-94; Feifel et al., 1973).

The process of dying in senile dementia may take a long time, but these patients cannot be reached. Such a psychological contact may be very meaningful, on the other hand, for persons who die of "old age," remaining conscious and oriented up to the end. There are certainly many patients in institutions for long-term care whose terminal period would be made more meaningful and easier by psychological terminal care along these lines; in these cases it is of minor importance which disease or diseases they happen to have.

WHICH PROFESSIONALS AND
IN WHICH SETTINGS

This approach to care of the dying has been developed by someone who happens to be a doctor, with qualifications as a psychiatrist as well as an oncologist. Those wishing to adopt the method naturally do not need to have this combination. Many of the requirements, which have been discussed earlier (p. 167), have more to do with personal characteristics than with professional qualifications. It is by no means sufficient, for instance, to be a doctor. Neither is training in psychiatry sufficient in itself. Neither medical nor psychiatric practice pays much attention at present to, for instance, existential problems. Some psychologists have more of the necessary theoretical training but lack familiarity with and experience of attending persons who are severely ill or dying.

Doctors, psychologists, social workers and nurses all seem to be in a position to apply this approach, provided they supplement their training. This supplement would be somewhat different for each group but should always include knowledge and experience of death and dying. Training and status are considerably less important, however, than the individual's motivation for working in close contact with dying persons.

The method which is described here has been integrated into an oncological department at a university teaching hospital. It can be used in various hospitals and in home care as well. Likewise, the psychological approach ought to be implemented in institutions such as hospices.

IS THERE SOMETHING SWEDISH ABOUT THE METHOD?

Friends abroad have now and then mentioned that my approach could be connected with Sweden especially. Frankly, I cannot see that point. A psychotherapeutic attitude is much more widespread, for instance, in the United States. Honestly and regrettably, "patient-centeredness" is not in any sense more typical for medical care in Sweden than elsewhere.

There is, on the other hand, a factor connected with the social policy of my country, which does greatly facilitate my work. As stated in the description of my professional setting, the patient does not pay for hospital care. This has many advantages for the implementation of my ideology and the method here described. It makes me feel free in relation to the patient and the patient is sure that I will stay by his side in accordance with his needs.

Chapter 11

Assessment of the Method

THE EVALUATION OF PSYCHOLOGICAL
TERMINAL CARE

The term method is frequently used in this book for the sake of brevity. A method may amount to a planned approach to the achievement of a goal, often the procurement of knowledge. In the case of therapeutic methods, for instance, the goal may be to influence a particular symptom or cure a disease. It seems natural to compare a method for terminal care with other therapeutic methods in care of the sick. One must, however, discuss whether this type of terminal care should be evaluated as treatment in the usual sense (see p. 177). Although it may be difficult to characterize in a few words, it is necessary to consider how this approach might be evaluated systematically.

In the evaluation of methods in the social and behavioral sciences, a distinction has been introduced recently between outcome research and process research.

Outcome research is about whether a particular measure or method does or does not have effects. Such an evaluation is strictly scientific, using controlled studies and measurements, often accompanied by statistical analysis of registered data.

Process research tries to identify the active agent in a measure or method, the way in which its effect is achieved and the course of the process. The literature on research and evaluation in psychotherapy has been rather contradictory and partly controversial but the distinction between these two lines has helped to clarify the picture. Process research, which is the more recent of the two, is attracting increasing interest in Sweden, as elsewhere.

When evaluating a method for care of the dying, one can aim to verify that an effect has been achieved (outcome research). The achievement can also be studied by means of comparisons with other methods. Attempts to use reports on clinical thanatology for such comparisons would meet with substantial difficulties, as discussed on pp. 8-10.

Finally, one can try to explore, i.e., observe, register and describe, what happens and try to catch relationships between those concerned and the implications of the method for them (process research). The present work is largely exploratory and the method is evaluated by observing and registering the effects on all concerned.

One difficulty in evaluating this method has to do with the fact that it is for dying persons. An inquiry in the spirit of outcome research—whether the goal of the method, to support and help dying persons, has been achieved—is out of the question for the simple reason that dying persons die. It would, nevertheless, be feasible during the course of dying to assess stages in this goal and to some extent verify such effects. Controlled studies would undoubtedly be complicated but in theory not impossible, even though I work in seclusion and cannot, for instance, accept the presence of observers. For process research, too, it is an obstacle that all my patients die and the significance for the dying of my activity must be evaluated largely indirectly.

A balanced evaluation is also rendered difficult or impossible by another aspect of work with the dying, an aspect that helps to explain why so many of us, doctors as well as laymen, avoid all discussion, study or consideration of the problem of death. As we are all involved in life and death, there is no one who can separate himself from the emotional aspect of dying and death—neither patient nor therapist, neither researcher nor those wishing to evaluate research. We shall all die; consequently, no one is objective or capable of viewing the problem from outside.

The difficulty is familiar from many other fields of research, although it is perhaps particularly apparent and inescapable when death is involved. A variety of methods and projects in medical care have to be evaluated by an engaged participant who must nevertheless try to maintain some distance in order to observe and describe. It would be neither meaningful nor fruitful to describe from outside a method, say, for tending the dying. The situation requires that one participate in the process. The matters to be described are the interaction, communication, dialogue and everything else that passes between two persons in a relationship. An attempt to remove the "human character" of one party would be to remove oneself from the core of the matter. The therapist is a not inconsiderable part of the total situation and hence an important component of the dying person's experience.

One possibility of assessing forms for terminal care is to use outside observers who try to evaluate how patients, relatives and staff experience the care. This approach has been used (Glaser & Strauss, 1965, 1968; Sudnow, 1967) but has its limitations. Such studies, often sociological in nature, can provide a valuable foundation, derived from relatively large numbers of patients, for describing general behavior. However, in order to catch psychological aspects, one has to come closer, which heightens the risk that the participation of an observer will influence the results.

As the nucleus of the present method is a confidential

relationship between patient and therapist, problems would be created by having an outside observer. The prospect of a "neutral" observer closely following a relationship between two persons, one of whom is slowly deteriorating and ultimately dies, directly conflicts with the conception and goal of my "ideology of care."

One can conceive of other, possibly less disturbing ways of obtaining information externally and objectively. Audiovisual aids are now being used more and more to register the verbal communication as well as the behavior of patient and therapist in a therapeutic contact. Such material can be an excellent foundation for discussions and instruction, but if it is used to evaluate the reality behind the recording, the risk of errors is greater than is usually realized. A severe disease or dying lasts some time and it is seldom possible to register and report the total course for the purpose of presenting a complete, balanced picture. The researcher must select the parts which he considers representative and in doing so he increases the risk of the results' being influenced by his subjective reactions to disease and death.

There are certain ethical aspects to consider when recording on sound or videotape. There is little difficulty, on the other hand, in obtaining permission from patients. This is usually given surprisingly—or rather disturbingly—easily. Dying persons are often so lonely that they will accept almost anything so long as someone will listen to them with fellow-feeling and interest. One has only to recall the well-known book by Kübler-Ross (1969) which is based on talks with dying persons in the presence of quite a few other people.

For my part, the idea of preserving the course of events in my work with dying persons is quite out of the question, as it would be incompatible with my entire approach to even suggest a tape or film recording. For one thing, my request to record our talks would obviously conflict with my promise that personal and emotional matters will not be divulged. For another, simply making such a request introduces an element of coercion. The situation of the patient and the nature of our contact often lead the patient to believe that he owes a debt of gratitude. Even if the patient is against the idea, he has difficulty in turning down a suggestion that he is liable to interpret—however neutrally one presents it—as being of interest for me or important for my activities as a thanatologist.

In the work described here, these considerations did not arise. When I started with psychological care of the dying and developed the present approach over a number of years, I had not thought of systematizing or publishing it. Consequently, there was never any question of planning a controlled study.

EFFECTS ON ALL CONCERNED

In this book I have in different ways conveyed as much as possible of the experience or of the process during my work. Here I will try to register and describe the reactions of all concerned. Those are the patients and the relatives, various categories of staff and people in general—including the reader —as well as the therapist.

Effect on the Patient

A great many memories come to mind when I try to distill how patients may have found me and our relationship. My subjective, general impression is that in these contacts I was of some benefit. By benefit I mean that the dying person was comforted by my presence, that our dialogue was meaningful and that the empathy I was able to show did something to reduce his anxiety. As the experience of dying is nearly always unwanted, feared and painful, we are concerned here with the extent to which a dire situation has been made more bearable.

My feeling that the contact was beneficial has to do with the quality of the dialogue, its increasing warmth, frankness and feeling of affinity. During our talks, many patients have indicated that our joint experience up to the end has been meaningful and valuable. Instances of this are the many times I was asked to come back and to do so soon, and the appeal from many patients that I would be there "when the time comes." To understand and assess such statements properly, they need to be seen in context. A number of examples have been quoted earlier in this book and there seems to be little point in adding others here.

Instead, one can ask whether my contact was harmful in any respect. This, too, is difficult to evaluate objectively and abstractly in retrospect. Obviously, there have been situations, exchanges and talks where I consider afterwards that I said the wrong thing, misinterpreted a signal or was not sufficiently alert to an appeal from the patient. It is equally clear that there have been psychodynamic situations which I have not understood or have handled incorrectly.

In contacts of this type, however, the question of good and bad is not as simple as this. To misinterpret a signal, for instance, is of course harmful; however, if the patient raises the matter again during that or a later session and I then understand him better and perhaps we exchange a smile of confirmation that the earlier mistake has not been repeated, it is conceivable that on the whole the incident has been beneficial. The same applies if the patient, having been disappointed or hurt, is able to take up the matter later in either a gentle, friendly manner or with obvious irritation that we both find natural.

Such situations have occurred and in evaluating them it is important to remember that they are never static. We always work with dimensions fluctuating between two poles. Misunderstandings as well as mutual understanding must be seen as components in a process. The inevitable, final nature of the outcome means that the question of benefit and harm is not quite the same as in other therapeutic contacts. The core of our dialogue is a shared experience of a process that the patient cannot escape from and the therapist participates in. A friendly gesture and a smile are just as much parts of the process as an aggressive reply or open displeasure. They contribute to complex dynamics against a background resonant with feelings and an awareness of the inevitable conclusion.

The appreciation and gratitude of a dying person are manifested most clearly in situations that are painful and trying and very personal for the patient. Since I am unwilling to relate everything that happens, this exposes me to the criticism that I am concealing just those matters which might be regarded as negative effects of my work. Having been in contact with a dying person for some time, however, it becomes evident whether the patient is finding the relationship fruitful or not. When discussing psychological terminal care, this experience has been confirmed by others who work in close contact with dying patients.

There is one respect in which I have definitely fulfilled a wish expressed by many patients, thereby perhaps being of some benefit. They have asked me to remember them and think of them from time to time.

Effect on Relatives

For the purpose of assessing effects of my work, it would be valuable to learn from relatives what they consider that the contact meant to the deceased, as well as how they themselves experienced my presence and my role. In reality, it is not easy to get separate answers to these two questions. Relatives have difficulty in distinguishing between their perception of the deceased's needs and wishes and the extent to which these were met, on the one hand, and their own view of my work, which may be colored by grief, anxiety and possibly jealousy, on the other. A lifetime of association with the deceased, memories of companionship and joy, of conflicts and separation, become mixed with the grief and sorrow and interfere with the assessment of events in the period when the patient was dying. In that I consistently broke off all contact with the relatives, the burden on them was undoubtedly great. It is difficult to tell how much was due to my participation and how much to the fact that the patient was dying.

Generalizing somewhat, I have observed over the years that the better the relationship between relatives and patient, the better the former were able, sooner or later, to accept my approach and appreciate it on the patient's and their own behalf. In families with emotional gaps, perennial quarrels and discord, the relatives were often irritated and suspicious of me and my way of working, especially when the contact was initiated just on account of problems with relatives. My knowledge of the emotional climate of the family rests on only a few observations and is colored in large measure by what I have learned from the patient. Even so, I find this observation valid.

Even when family relationships are balanced and harmonious, my contact with the patient is unquestionably a difficulty for the relatives. They may appreciate that a stranger is prepared to talk with the patient about disease and death, sharing his anxiety, suffering and pain, but this is also liable to arouse their jealousy, just as bringing in an outsider is liable to increase their feeling of helplessness and inadequacy. The therapist may be regarded as a "stand-in" who is needed because the relatives have failed in some respect. The need for a "new friend" may be difficult to understand and even hurt the relatives. They may also want to turn to me to discuss aspects of what is happening and obtain advice about answering the dying person's questions or complying with his wishes. My refusal to respond in these profoundly human and understandable contexts is bound to arouse aggressiveness, anxiety and disappointment. It may also be difficult to realize that they are being discussed with an outsider, who alone hears what the patient has experienced and suffered.

In my experience, few relatives seemed to be displeased, when they tried to see the matter *from the patient's point of view*. On the contrary, most of them expressed appreciation of my work for the patient. They conveyed to me, at our first talk as well as indirectly in various ways and sometimes after the patient's death, that they understood my aim and felt that the patient had received valuable support.

Turning instead to how the relatives experienced my work *from their own point of view,* a distinction that, as mentioned, is difficult and partly artificial, it can be noted that an occasional family found my presence burdensome or was even against it. As indicated earlier, these relatives mostly had difficulties and tensions among themselves. Many relatives have understood my role and seen that it benefited them as well. They found the dying person easier to talk with and be with up to the end and realized that this was because difficult problems became less prominent as the patient discussed them with me. After the patient's death, several relatives have thus indicated that their burden and anxiety during the final phase had proved easier to bear than they had expected because during our talk the dying person had defused his conflicts with them.

During talks quite a long time afterwards with relatives of the five patients described in Chapter 5, I met a very favorable reaction to my work. I asked whether I might publish the case histories that appear in this book and in giving their permission they often indicated that they considered my work was beneficial, that the deceased had talked to them appreciatively about me, that I had really understood the deceased's personality, and that they hoped my work would lead to an improvement in hospital care of the dying.

Talks with other relatives of the 38 patients have taught me that relatives may be uncomfortable or opposed to meeting me for many reasons without necessarily being displeased with my work. For instance, two relatives whom I encountered in other contexts said that they had avoided me because they had remarried and assumed that I would "side with the deceased" and perhaps condemn this.

The grief reaction of relatives should be included in an assessment of effects, but in most cases I never heard about its subsequent course and these aspects can therefore not be analyzed here.

A very few relatives have gotten in touch and asked me to give them psychiatric support. If I understood them correctly, they had been favorably impressed with my work with the deceased and wanted to continue with me for that reason. It is debatable whether this would be suitable psychiatrically or in view of my agreement with the patient. In my opinion, it would be more advisable for them to get in touch with another psychologist or psychiatrist.

When using this method for terminal care, it would be desirable for another psychiatrist to look after relatives right from the time when the therapist starts his contact with the patient. This independent psychiatrist could then follow the family afterwards and provide support as they work through their grief. By systemizing experiences from such parallel work with dying and their relatives, one would be in a better position to judge the magnitude of the burden on relatives and thereby assess whether indications for the method need to be modified.

Reactions of the Hospital Staff

The work done in hospitals on behalf of terminal care has often been criticized in the current debate (Feigenberg & Fulton, 1976a, b). When improvements are suggested or, as in the present case, an attempt is made to introduce a special approach to care of the dying, the reactions among hospital staff are of two completely different kinds. A call for a greater commitment is received skeptically and unwillingly by a majority, and is adopted rather uncritically and optimistically by a minority.

The hospital hierarchy is such that the effects on the staff of a particular approach can hardly be described unless one takes each category separately.

Doctors. The reactions of the doctors should be seen in the light of their general attitude and that of other hospital personnel to dying and death. The following comments represent my own views and experiences. No attempt has been made to obtain the views of my colleagues, for instance, by discussing my work directly with them. A systematic study by a third party would have been desirable but, as I originally had no intention of publishing my experiences, this was not arranged.

The picture that crystallizes out my personal impression, from direct talks as well as indirect reactions and statements, is roughly as follows. Some doctors have expressed appreciation and a favorable reaction to my work, while others have been indifferent or even opposed to it. At one end of the scale, there are the doctors who willingly supported my work, knowing about and accepting my special approach. At the other extreme, there are a few colleagues whose reactions were definitely unfavorable.

When I first started using this method, it happened that one or two patients were discharged after our contact had been established and against my will. It is legitimate to question my interpretation of such an incident, but in some cases it was evident that the doctor clearly realized that this measure placed a severe strain both on the patient and on me. There have also been ironical and condescending remarks about my activity from some colleagues, in most cases to the effect that it is a waste of time or hardly ethical to burrow into the thoughts and feelings of the dying patient.

Disapproving doctors or nurses have not infrequently drawn my attention to any number of risks which a close contact could involve for the dying patient, for me and for the hospital as a whole. While some of their fears may be justified, they chiefly illustrate some current attitudes toward terminal care.

The positive and negative reactions to work of this type will be familiar to many of those engaged in clinical thanatology. It is perhaps more important to draw attention to a third position, which constitutes the reaction of a majority of doctors to my approach: *complete silence*. Note that these are patients whom I have managed for a considerable time, coming and going on the wards, borrowing records to keep up with the somatic course, altering medication and naturally encountering all categories of ward staff all the time. Even so, many of the doctors who were responsible for the somatic care never commented on my activity, either at the time or after the patient's death.

The last point is not quite true. I do sometimes hear a comment, shortly after a patient's death, from those responsible for his care, but from this silent majority it is the only opinion that reaches me. It comes in guises such as, "It was best that way," "Good thing it's over," "It was best like that for everyone."

Although these are positive statements, their implications are dubious. What happened was obviously not "best." We shall all die but for this particular person it might just as well have happened 20 years later. Seen from the patient's viewpoint and considering his life as a whole, perhaps it would have been better had he died earlier or lived longer.

It makes one wonder when hospital staff believe they know when and how things are "best" when fundamentally they are so extremely "bad." One wonders to whom "best for everyone" refers. Could it be the relatives? Despite all their ambivalent relationships, the relatives are usually grieved or broken-hearted; they, too, often say that it was best that way, generally in an attempt to comfort themselves and each other but perhaps also as a reflection of ambivalent feelings.

But in what way is it "best" when the doctor says this? Perhaps it does ultimately refer to the hospital staff as a whole, implying that it is all over for now and one can take a break. I may be wrong, but these comments do seem to reflect the emotional quality which hospital care in general has at present when it comes to care of the dying. At all events, having devoted oneself to the patient in accordance with my approach and having gotten to know him as a person, it is difficult to accept "it was best that way" as the sole comment during the whole of this period.

A great many patients have died at Radiumhemmet during these years without anyone contacting me. I am not aware of the reasons for this or the deliberations that may have taken place in the individual case. But it is noteworthy that a substantial number of patients were referred to me from certain wards, while none was ever referred from others.

In summary, it is my general impression that the doctors who came into contact with the activity described here generally shielded themselves and took very little interest in it. Of all the doctors who were attached to Radiumhemmet in the years I have worked there, only a limited number have displayed a real interest in my activity.

Nurses. In general, when terminally ill patients have been under my care at Radiumhemmet, I have tried to engage the nurses in the psychological care of dying patients. The nurse can take part in talks with the patient if this appears suitable and she can often take over part of the contact with relatives.

In the patient-centered contacts described here, the nurses were in a completely different situation. My agreement with the patient that our contact should be completely confidential applied even to the nurses. Their participation in the control of pain (see p. 134) was an exception in this respect, but the nurses had no means of knowing what really passed between me and the patient and consequently may have felt left out. Their work may have been facilitated, on the other hand, in that I was there to discuss difficult questions with the patient and share his anxiety.

An extra burden as a result of my work may have arisen because it is agreed that patients with whom I have this special contact will be allowed to remain at Radiumhemmet even if the usual routine would have indicated a transfer. This means that the ward has to cope with an additional number of terminal cases. Some patients were referred to me just because the staff found them a strain or provoking and in such cases a patient whom the staff found difficult had to remain on the ward.

Another difficulty arose when a patient was displeased with me and communicated his disappointment and aggressiveness to the nurse. She then felt that, if she could talk about this with me, not only would she avoid an awkward intermediate position but she would also help the patient. Not being able to do this must have been a strain.

An important means of diminishing these difficulties lies in the information that the nurses received about my approach.

If possible, I talked with the nurses on the ward each time I started a contact with a patient. It was not always possible, however, to keep the nurses well-informed and there is a gap between understanding a certain approach in theory and putting it into practice in a variety of specific situations, which in this case are always associated with anxiety and tension.

My general impression is that the nurses were predominantly in favor of my work. Many indicated—by a nod or a friendly smile in passing or by a spontaneous appreciative phrase—that my visit would be good for the patient and that they themselves agreed with my approach. Patients frequently told me that they had discussed me, my work and what it meant with the nurses, whose responses and reactions as related by the patient revealed that many of them had given appropriate, shrewd support. They had understood intuitively what I was aiming at and assisted my work indirectly.

At times, the situation became complex and difficult for a nurse to bear, resulting in signs of irritation or ill-will. I was, moreover, presumably unaware of many of their reactions, feelings and thoughts about my work with the patients. In order to reduce these difficulties, besides providing information about my approach, I tried to meet the staff after the patient's death in order to discuss and analyze any questions and conflicts (see p. 161).

If this approach is to be used in the future, it is definitely important that, while the terminal contact is in progress, the nurses are given emotional support and an opportunity to work through their feelings with the aid of a competent outsider.

Other staff. Most categories of staff do not have a clearly defined role when it comes to care of the dying. Assistant nurses, aides and night attendants would seem to have specific, clearly defined roles and tasks in practical care of the sick. It is expected that they will refer all questions and difficulties of patients and relatives to the nurses or doctors, particularly about such "difficult" matters as dying and death. It is now generally realized that they do not strictly adhere to these rules. Indeed, it is inconceivable that two people could meet frequently over a considerable period in a situation where one of them is fatally ill and the other calls to clean up, wash the floor, hand out and collect meal-trays or have the sole task of sitting by the sick-bed, without mentioning the main event in the room. This is all the more unlikely as these staff members appear to be those who are most prepared to really talk with the patient. Many are elderly, with experience of what life may have in store.

The chance of assessing how *assistant nurses, aides* and *night attendants* have experienced my activity was unfortunately limited. My contacts with this group, although incomplete, leave the general impression that my work was considered beneficial. Several have conveyed a feeling of warm solidarity. I have many memories of assistants or night attendants who greeted me warmly before leaving when I entered the room, which was the agreed procedure when I had this special contact with the patient. I had the feeling of being welcomed and an impression that the staff member shared the patient's anticipation and favorable attitude. If this could not be expressed by an enfeebled patient, it was conveyed by the aide's manner of greeting me and the quick smile of mutual understanding she exchanged with the patient.

When I attended a patient's funeral, the company often included some of the staff from the ward and it happened that one of them would come up to me, exchange a few words, and indicate that she wanted to stand beside me during the funeral in order to mark a fellow-feeling. This seemed natural as we were both taking farewell of someone who had been close to us.

Social workers have qualified training that includes psychology, but in Sweden they regrettably seldom participate in the actual care of dying persons. As far as I can tell, they were favorably disposed and, whenever social workers had contact with my patients, they followed my intentions and thereby facilitated my work.

Physiotherapists have a well-defined task in care of the sick. Many severely ill patients have close physical contact daily with a physiotherapist and naturally strike up a relationship.

Physiotherapists have often asked for instruction in terminal care or assistance with specific problems relating to this and they have also gotten in touch with me to relate or ask something about one of my patients.

Sometimes a physiotherapist becomes very close to a patient and, just because the physiotherapist is not considered to be one of those who is "managing the disease," the patient is often able to express fears and anxiety about death, besides discussing personal difficulties in general.

> A severely ill man who was referred to me relatively late in the course of his disease proved difficult to get close to. There were no relatives and he appeared lonely and full of anxiety. Something remained unspoken between us and just then I could not find a reasonable way of resolving the difficulty. One day the physiotherapist, who had been giving the patient about a half-hour's treatment daily, got in touch with me quite unexpectedly. She had observed and understood the patient while talking with him during the treatment and she now informed me that he was homosexual. Many pieces of the puzzle then fell into place and became comprehensible. The physiotherapist either did not know or did not bother about my special rules for these patients; she was concerned for the patient, liked him and considered it important that I knew what she had to tell.

Department of Psychiatry. The emphasis I place on the psychological aspect of terminal care could perhaps be taken to mean that these ideas are generally accepted in psychiatry or in psychiatric care in Sweden or at least at the psychiatric department to which I belong. It should be noted, therefore, that attitudes toward death and toward care of the dying are very much the same in psychiatry as in the rest of medical care. The personnel have the same basic training and one encounters the same attitudes, often even the same uncertainty and bewilderment, when confronted with terminally ill patients.

In respect to this study, I had to contact the Department of Psychiatry mostly when severely ill or dying patients needed psychiatric hospital care. Generally, I have had difficulty in obtaining a bed for such patients. While the Department of Psychiatry at Karolinska Hospital is often overcrowded, with considerable pressure from patients in need of acute psychiatric care, I do have the impression that there was an emotional resistance to patients in the terminal phase, which in itself is understandable. On those few occasions when I wanted to arrange a bed for a patient, this took considerable time and much persuasion.

It is, of course, true that the staff at a psychiatric clinic are neither accustomed to dying patients nor trained to handle them. On the other hand, it is inevitable that even severely ill and dying persons may need psychiatric hospital care. I occupy an intermediate position here and sometimes feel that the emotional difficulties are transferred in part to affects against me as the perceived cause of an unaccustomed, trying situation for the psychiatric staff. This is similar to the irritation I sometimes encounter on an oncologic ward if a patient is psychologically deviant. I may then receive an emotional demand to transfer the patient at once to the psychiatric clinic, even though the patient is under treatment and the psychological symptoms only moderate.

This attitude is more in evidence on some wards than on others, in both the psychiatric and the oncologic sector. In general, however, it can be said that psychiatrists and psychiatric staff are about as tolerant, or rather intolerant, of severe somatic diseases and terminality as are their somatic colleagues and staff of deviant psychological behavior.

Effect on Other Patients

Little appears to have been written about the part played by other patients in the psychological events surrounding those who are severely ill and dying. My experience definitely indicates that they often have a large and sometimes an overwhelming influence on the dying person's experiences. Patients can give one another invaluable support and encouragement but may equally well be a source of anxiety and resignation. The latter is particularly noticeable when another patient dies of something which the patient interprets as the same disease or complication as his own.

My patients have often told me what other patients meant to them, the ways in which they received support and comfort or admired how another patient bore his suffering. At times they have also expressed anxiety, aggressiveness or ill-will as a reaction to what other patients have done or said.

Co-patients have sometimes conveyed thoughts and feelings that are relevant here in the course of my daily rounds or during chance meetings in the hospital. Some have wanted to indicate that my visit to a particular patient is a good thing: "He badly needs it" or "it makes her so happy." Others have made it clear that they certainly do not need me or my assistance, others again that they hope on the contrary I will be there later should they need me.

Without conducting any systematic study, I conclude, from what I have heard from my own patients and from the comments of co-patients, that the mere existence of a person devoted to the dying and the possibility of such a confidential, psychological contact, if needed, have a deep impact on the other patients on a ward.

Reactions From the Public

When meeting the general public in discussions after lectures or articles about aspects of death and dying, I often get reactions which are specifically related to my patient-centered approach for care of dying. What I have picked up on many such occasions is at one extreme a somewhat solemn respect for a person who dares to come that near to the dying. The other extreme involves accusations of my dubious motives, indicating my "morbid curiosity."

Many tend to comment upon my special way of handling the relatives. Here, again, some call me downright cruel, while others need to express that had they known earlier of this approach, their father's or wife's death could have been altogether different.

As a whole, I more often meet extreme attitudes to my work than more balanced considerations. The same goes for hospital administrators, clergy and even doctors, who, in a public setting, can be looked upon as part of the public and voice the so-called public opinion. Some almost contemplate trying to stop me, while others claim that all dying people should be entitled to this kind of care. I object equally to both of these opinions.

Readers. Whatever we read, irrespective of the subject, affects us intellectually and emotionally. If the subject has little to do with the reader's own interests or occupation, the emotional effect is presumably slight. Other subjects are of more general concern and no one can dissociate himself from them. These include life, love and a few more. Death in any event leaves no one unmoved, while most people find it predominantly alarming and frightening. Consequently, readers undoubtedly react emotionally to this book and to much of what is said in it. This is not, in fact, an unintended effect on my part. The crucial point is whether the individual reader himself is aware that he reacts emotionally.

Reactions of the Therapist

An evaluation of this approach to care of the dying must include the therapist. His importance obviously varies with the kind of method for terminal care but this person is always relevant to some extent and in many contexts highly significant. In my opinion, one should try to report one's own impressions and also the difficulties of making an "objective" assessment of an approach in which personality is inevitably a major component.

It is given to few to really fathom their own emotions. Still fewer, e.g., Freud and Kierkegaard, have truly made a contribution to important knowledge and insights by means of self-analysis.

Some refuse to recognize that they have attitudes which influence their observations; others consider that they "allow" for these. But if one is to allow for personal attitudes, conceptions, feelings and so on, it is necessary to know about them in detail. How many people can have objective, exact knowledge and insight about their own feelings concerning dying and death?

No one can, in fact, regard the problem of death objectively and externally. There are many indications (see p. 218) that we cannot enter into and comprehend "emotionally" what it involves, how it feels not to exist—to be dead. No one denies explicitly that we shall all die, but each one of us has fantasies, explanations, secret hopes or firmly rooted religious or philosophical attitudes toward death. These are bound to influence anyone who thinks, talks and writes about death and there is no reason why I should be an exception.

It is clear that *psychological factors* play a part in the choice of a particular occupation or line of work. One wonders whether thanatologists in general have some special attitudes toward death. Attempts have been made to investigate this, without reaching any definite conclusions (Mahoney & Kyle, 1976; Burton, 1978).

I am only partly aware of the innermost reasons for my own choice of occupation. Personal experience of relatives' illnesses contributed. Having worked for some years with psychological care of cancer patients, I became increasingly conscious of the special problems associated with death and the responsibility of the medical profession for care of the dying.

Two factors in particular led me to develop a special approach to care of dying cancer patients. One was a reaction against the denial, avoidance and rejection of dying patients that one encounters in hospital care. This made it necessary to investigate the problem thoroughly in order to give my criticism weight. In time I arrived at the ideology of care described here, which focuses on the personality and individuality of the patient. The other factor was a conscious desire to develop as personal a contact as possible with dying patients. A close individual and psychological contact with suffering persons that excludes everyone around us apparently fits something in my personal makeup.

An intense, private psychological contact with a person whom one accompanies up to the end is bound to have *psychological effects* on oneself, too. Work with the dying according to this method is demanding and emotionally burdensome. As indicated earlier, I do not consider that I can manage more than two patients concurrently with this method. I find it difficult to present my personal experiences in connection with individual patients but my feelings have been described earlier in this book, both directly and indirectly. I presumably have many reactions and emotions of which I am not myself aware.

Identification with the patient always arises, as described earlier, in a close contact with a dying person, though to varying degrees. Some patients and some situations have naturally involved me more than others. When following a dying person closely, one is bound to deal consciously and subconsciously with what the course implies and where it leads. I know that it is the patient and not myself who is going to die and can therefore maintain a certain distance, but one cannot dismiss the thought that this is my future, too. The thought of my own death forces itself upon me.

The imminent death of the patient elicits my grief and this feeling increases as our relationship becomes closer. In principle, however, this is not the same as grieving for someone with whom one has been close for many years, or with whom one has shared parts or the whole of one's life. Many thoughts and feelings naturally arise, consciously and subconsciously, during the course of a contact. I may feel anxiety at the thought of the patient, but the anxiety may also concern me. Aggressiveness may be aroused—it may seem that a patient is deceiving me: Even though I have invested so much emotional energy in him, he is still going to die and leave me. During a talk I may not have understood, not been sufficiently attuned to a patient, or inadequate in some other way; all this gives me guilt feelings now.

A general observation concerning my feelings about a patient's imminent death presumably illustrates an aspect of my feelings and needs in contacts with patients. As long as we maintain a dialogue that we both find meaningful and full of interest, even though it may vary in intensity, I find the emotional burden quite bearable. I have had no difficulty, for instance, in managing other patients, who were not dying, at the same time. It is when the patient becomes partly or completely unconscious that I find the burden heaviest. When I visit a patient, with whom I have shared innumerable thoughts and problems, and can only stand by the bed, getting no response when I say his name, it is then that I experience grief tinged with helplessness.

There have, of course, been moments when a contact has felt almost overwhelming. At some subconscious level, I hope against hope that the person with whom I have become so close is somehow going to survive. When it suddenly becomes clear that this irrational hope has no foundation and I realize quite clearly that the patient is dying, grief may result but also a wish that death will not be long in coming. This is not always just to spare the patient but also because I, too, wish to be spared. Presumably, it is such a feeling deep inside that causes me to react violently in turn when doctors and nurses assure me, after the patient's death, that it was "best that way" (p. 198).

A personal, wholehearted human relationship with a dying person is frequently a heavy burden but it is also—and this unfortunately is not generally recognized in care of the sick— deeply involving, meaningful and rewarding.

I have been asked by quite a few colleagues, as well as by others, whether I myself am afraid to die, whether I experience death-anxiety or how I view my own death. These persons have often revealed indirectly that they consider these questions private and personal. In many cases, the question has been intended to expose and trip me up.

People seem to think that those who want to launch thanatology as a field for both theoretical and clinical research are emotional robots. They believe, or hope, that in some way we are free from ordinary human feelings or protected from death-anxiety through our work. Of course we are not and that is one of the reasons why we are thanatologists.

Chapter 12

Conclusions

In this book I have attempted to convey an ideology of care which I have tried to put into practice in psychological care of the dying. The aim of this "method" for a psychological contact is to share another person's condition of being a dying individual, a condition that is unique for each one of us, yet inevitable. The means for this is a dialogue, as open as possible, in which innermost thoughts and feelings find expression. The therapist, who knows that the patient is dying, must nevertheless be able to side with him in his "conception of immortality." Although aware that death is unavoidable, he must be prepared to revolt together with the dying person or share the fantasies and hopes, as well as the anxiety and ambivalent feelings, that are aroused in the patient by the approaching threat.

One of the purposes of writing this book has been to *present a method* for psychological terminal care. To this end I have described the same process and same events from different angles and at different levels.

When it comes to *evaluating effects of the method,* it must be noted that there is no means of knowing whether my approach helped the dying person. This presentation has presumably indicated that I not only hope but consider it probable that my work was to some extent beneficial. The essential point is not so much whether the method had an effect; more important is to describe what took place and how all concerned may have experienced my approach towards contacts with dying persons. Those concerned also include myself, as a person involved in the terminal contact I wish to describe. I have deliberately attempted to enter into a process and at the same time keep a certain distance in order to observe, register and describe what happens.

Work of this type may pose the question: What is it that achieves the effects? It may be the therapist's personality, the method with all its technical rules, quite different factors or possibly a mixture of them all. The answer to this question is decisive for whether others can learn to use the method.

Seen from my position, this is an extreme method. But the approach was chosen to some extent deliberately as a reaction against the health service's tendency to deny or gloss over the psychological aspect of dying. Although the method as a whole may be applicable only in certain situations, there are many aspects that are valid in clinical thanatology in general.

The study of effects on those concerned indicates that the method also has drawbacks. It imposes a considerable burden on relatives. To determine whether this is so great that the approach should be modified in this respect, controlled studies would have to be undertaken with psychiatrists or psychologists in touch with the relatives concurrently with the terminal contact. It can also be concluded that if a method of this type is to be used, the staff will need both thorough information about its principles and adequate psychological support.

My work to support dying persons on the psychological level has yielded some insights and experience. As a contribution to the *psychology of dying,* there is my experience that the most characteristic feature in the course of dying is its varying and multidimensional emotional content. Some such dimensions relevant during dying are explored and discussed. Dying is a process that lasts for a certain time, ending with death; however, I could not find that it was divisible into clear-cut phases. If one tries to come close and observe without theoretical preconceptions, it will be found that the psychological chain of events is extremely irregular and chaotic. Consequently, the therapeutic task is precisely to have the strength to share this chaos and yet maintain some stability or security.

The health service and perhaps to some extent the general public regard or would like to regard dying as a uniform, uneventful process, so that all dying persons need is basic care. This attitude does not seem to have been greatly altered so far by the powerful evidence to the contrary from clinical thanatology. The extent to which psychological needs are ignored in terminal care struck me more strongly than I had expected during my work with dying persons. These patients have a boundless need to convey to someone who they are and who they have been during their lives, to relate their disappointments and defeats, their hopes and successes, and to share all that they are now experiencing while dying and their fantasies about what is to come. In the light of my experience, it is unimaginative and cruel to deny people this or, as happens at present, to let most of those who die in an institution die alone.

For *practical medical care* this study has thus strengthened my conviction that there is an enormous need for psychological work in care of the dying. Although the method described here has only a limited field of use, there is not the least chance at present of providing terminal care of this type for even a few of the patients for whom it is indicated.

It is necessary in this context to discuss terminal care as a whole. In view of this experience from a highly specialized method for psychological terminal care, developed and practiced in a conventional oncological institution, one is made starkly aware of the health service's total lack of explicit standards and goals for the care of dying persons. I do not consider that, even if circumstances permitted, a method such as the one described here should be practiced generally in health service by specialists in terminal care. This would simply lower the psychological quality of the health service in general. All personnel must be trained in psychological terminal care. But this requires that in the first place one appropriately discuss and agree about the goal for and structure of this terminal care. The use of the method in question must be restricted to specific indications and applied when appropriately trained clinical thanatologists are available.

For *psychiatry* I consider that my work with dying cancer patients has taught me that the appropriate framework for psychological terminal care is a dynamic psychiatry based on psychoanalytical thinking, but free from dogmatic ties to a rigid conceptual apparatus, and with an open mind about *existential problems.*

APPENDICES

Appendix I

Survey of the Thanatological Literature

People have thought and written about death for as long as they have thought and written at all in the history of mankind. Death features in the sacred writings of all religions, its meaning is interpreted and people are instructed how to meet it. All through the ages, major philosophical works have wrestled with death or taken it as their starting point. It is a cornerstone in all social systems and political doctrines.

The literature underlying present-day thanatology comes mainly from the fields of psychology and sociology and goes back a mere half-century. It is difficult to say who made the first contribution. A suitable starting point, if one concentrates on the psychological aspect of thanatology and focuses on the dying individual, is what Freud wrote about death.

FREUD'S THANATOLOGY

Freud's works are strewn with observations relating to death but there are two in particular that have played a decisive part in reflections about death in the present century (Gifford, 1969):

1) The concept of unconscious immortality
2) The concept "death instinct"

Unconscious immortality. In 1915, in the midst of the first world war, Freud wrote an essay entitled *Zeitgemässes über Krieg und Tod* ("Thoughts for the Times on War and Death").

> It is indeed impossible to imagine our own death; and whenever we attempt to do so we can perceive that we are in fact still present as spectators. Hence the psycho-analytic school could venture on the assertion that at bottom no one believes in his own death, or, to put the same thing in another way, that in the unconscious every one of us is convinced of his own immortality.

In Freud's view, no one can really conceive of his own death, that is, really imagine what it means not to exist. As a result, most people think of death as something that comes from outside, a thing that afflicts us or is the work of someone or something. We are therefore constantly looking for this something, that is, the cause of death.

Freud also elaborated the fundamental distinction between "my own death," that of "my enemy" and that of "my friend." The quotation above concerns "our own death." On the subject of our "enemy's" death Freud writes:

> On the other hand, for strangers and for enemies we do acknowledge death, and consign them to it quite as readily and unhesitatingly as did primaeval man. There is, it is true, a distinction here which will be pronounced decisive as far as real life is concerned. Our unconscious does not carry out the killing; it merely thinks it and wishes it. But it would be wrong so completely to undervalue this psychical reality as compared with factual reality. It is significant and momentous enough. In our unconscious impulses we daily and hourly get rid of anyone who stands in our way, of anyone who has offended or injured us.

The death of our enemy pleases us and at least subconsciously we have often wished for it. It therefore gives us satisfaction, but we may also have guilt-feelings.

In the same essay Freud writes about the death of our "friend":

> With the exception of only a very few situations, there adheres to the tenderest and most intimate of our love-relations

a small portion of hostility which can excite an unconscious death-wish. But this conflict due to ambivalence does not now, as it did then, lead to the doctrine of the soul and to ethics, but to neurosis, which affords us deep insight into normal mental life as well.

This is developed in another passage:

What released the spirit of enquiry in man was not the intellectual enigma, and not every death, but the conflict of feeling at the death of loved yet alien and hated persons. Of this conflict of feeling psychology was the first offspring. Man could no longer keep death at a distance, for he had tasted it in his pain about the dead; but he was nevertheless unwilling to acknowledge it, for he could not conceive of himself as dead. So he devised a compromise: he conceded the fact of his own death as well, but denied it the significance of annihilation—a significance which he had had no motive for denying where the death of his enemy was concerned. It was beside the dead body of someone he loved that he invented spirits, and his sense of guilt at the satisfaction mingled with his sorrow turned these new-born spirits into evil demons that had to be dreaded. The (physical) changes brought about by death suggested to him the division of the individual into a body and a soul—originally several souls. In this way his train of thought ran parallel with the process of disintegration which sets in with death. His persisting memory of the dead became the basis for assuming other forms of existence and gave him the conception of a life continuing after apparent death.

When our friend, perhaps a person we love, dies, we go through a complicated psychological process because emotional relationships are always ambivalent. Unsullied love is rare, and so is pure hate. By the same token, our feelings for a friend are tinged, on a certain level or in a particular sense, by animosity. We feel misunderstood, insufficiently loved or appreciated. Besides eliciting grief, his death may therefore give us feelings of guilt, malice or relief.

Freud's description of our subconscious sense of immortality is a central motive in thanatological thought. It has been discussed and re-interpreted by many writers. It is termed "the primary paradox" by Weisman (1972), whose book *On Dying and Denying* starts from this paradox. Lifton (1973, 1976) reformulates the problem by showing that we have a fantasy about immortality, which we give a symbolic content. He argues that we have an idea that life continues and that this is expressed in the process of symbolization that he regards as one of man's fundamental psychological characteristics. Lifton considers that on the subconscious level we are neither convinced of our immortality nor sure that we shall die, adopting instead a position somewhere between these extremes. This generates an inner need to create and develop images of a symbolic continuation of life.

The psychoanalytical school has been criticized—justifiably on the whole—for paying relatively little attention to the problem of death in clinical work. Neither has psychoanalysis been used very much in the treatment of dying patients, though it is admittedly about the only school of psychology-psychiatry to have contributed substantially to an understanding of the problem of dying.

This lack of interest in therapy for the dying and in dealing with the problem of death in an analysis may have to do with the anxiety which work with the dying provokes in us all, psychoanalysts included (Weisman, 1977). Many writers (Wahl, 1958; Rosenthal, 1963; Stern, 1968) have found the cause in Freud's strong emphasis on our subconscious belief in immortality. As a result, psychoanalysts and psychiatrists have left questions about death to philosophers and others. Freud was misinterpreted as meaning that any interest in immortality amounted to a denial of death, whereas in fact he championed the cause of a frank, direct approach to death. The essay quoted here ends with a famous adaption of an old saying: "If you want to endure life, prepare yourself for death."

Death instinct. Around 1919 Freud developed the idea of two "Triebe" (translated somewhat unfortunately as instincts): "Lebenstriebe" and "Todestriebe." These are seen as fundamental and overriding principles that regulate the function of all organisms (Freud, 1920).

It is not clear how Freud's thoughts about death, related above, are to be reconciled with the conception of "Todestriebe" and how they can be combined in clinical work. Opinions on this have differed widely. Eissler (1955) completely accepts the concept of "death instinct" and appears to use it in his assessment of clinical situations. Others have completely denied the existence of this phenomenon and consider it quite unusable (Fromm-Reichmann, 1959). The underlying theoretical discussion is complex (Hamilton, 1976; Wallace, 1976) and this is not the place to go into it. It is worth mentioning, however, that contemporary French psychoanalytic thinking has given the death instinct a new interpretation, which may become fruitful (Laplanche, 1970).

CONTEMPORARY THANATOLOGICAL WRITING

The *psychological* contribution to writings on thanatology had at first, as mentioned, a predominantly psychoanalytical orientation. Since then, however, the classical school of psychoanalysis has done little to further discussion about death. More has been done by researchers who have a psychodynamic orientation but are independent of psychoanalysis. Psychological systematizers with an eclectic outlook have undertaken valuable thanatological research, often together or parallel with sociological groups, rendering thanatology relatively independent of any one psychiatric line.

Leaving aside recent methodological developments in behavioral therapy and the competition between this and the psychodynamic school, one would like to speculate about the extent to which behavioral therapy and its application might be of value in contacts with persons who are dying. The literature where this is discussed (Preston, 1973; Whitman & Lukes, 1975) is not very convincing.

Sociological studies of dying and death, many of them undertaken together with psychological or anthropological groups, have considerably enriched thanatology (Fulton, 1976).

Philosophy has always been interested in death (Choron, 1963, 1964) and questions about life and its meaning, the content of death (Kaufmann, 1959) and the nature of anxiety have been primary concerns in *existentialist* thought. Thanatology has been greatly influenced by the combined effect of existential theories and dynamic psychology (Weisman, 1965).

A systematic review of the literature behind today's thanatology lies outside the scope of this book. Thanatology is developing rapidly at present, extending the area of its contacts with other disciplines such as oncology and internal medicine, or economics and demography. By way of a background to clinical thanatology, which is based on general theoretical thanatology, some basic works are introduced very briefly below. Some of these volumes are anthologies and contain the most pertinent aspects of contemporary thanatological thought and research. For a wider view of this field, the reader is referred to a bibliography that contains almost 4000 titles (Fulton, 1977a) or a new critically annotated bibliography (Simpson, 1979).

BASIC WORKS ON THANATOLOGY

EISSLER, K. *The Psychiatrist and the Dying Patient*, 1955, Reprinted in a pocket edition, 1969.

This is a pioneer work on what the psychiatrist can do in care of the dying. It has meant a great deal for persons, including myself, whose work centers on terminal care. The author is a psychoanalyst and the reader needs to be acquainted with the conceptual apparatus of psychoanalysis. The book is made up of three parts: a broad introduction to theoretical thanatology, excellent descriptions of three patients who died with cancer and a conclusion with a discussion of euthanasia and orthothanasia.

FEIFEL, H. (ED.) *The Meaning of Death*, 1959

This first anthology to appear deals with many thanatological questions and played a major part in the development of contemporary thanatology. Many of the contributions are very well-written by prominent researchers in various fields. This book has now been followed by the excellent *New Meanings of Death* (Feifel, 1977).

FULTON, R. (ED.) *Death and Identity,* 1965. New edition 1976.

Fulton is a sociologist who has written alone or in collaboration about many aspects of death and grief. This book is an anthology with highly competent linking comments by the editor. Its new edition is very informative and comprehensive.

HINTON, J. *Dying,* 1967.

A brief, but comprehensive and balanced account of questions in thanatology by a single author, who is a professor of psychiatry in London. A very good introduction to the field.

KUBLER-ROSS, E. *On Death and Dying,* 1969.

This book, by a psychiatrist, has become a best-seller all over the world and been of enormous importance through the interest it has aroused, even among the general public, in practical questions to do with clinical thanatology.

The strength of the book lies in the verbatim extracts from some of the many talks that the author, despite opposition from doctors, has had with dying persons. She manages to convey the emotional gain from these talks for all concerned. There are some theoretical views on thanatology which are debatable and controversial.

BRIM, O. G., JR. et. al. (EDS.) *The Dying Patient,* 1970.

This anthology contains many important works on clinical thanatology. It focuses on the dying person but also deals at length with the opinions and problems of the professional groups engaged in care of the sick.

KASTENBAUM, R. & AISENBERG, R. *The Psychology of Death,* 1972. Abbreviated edition, 1976.

Kastenbaum, a professor of psychology, has worked for many years on aging and death. This is unquestionably a standard work, a penetrating and fundamental discussion of the psychology of death. For those who only want to read one book about thanatology, this must be the choice.

WEISMAN, A. *On Dying and Denying*, 1972.

The author, a psychoanalyst and existentialist, is a thinker and researcher of impressive personal integrity. For many years he has led a large research project on dying patients, chiefly cancer patients. His findings, descriptions and definitions are of great importance for anyone wishing to become familiar with psychological care of the dying.

SHNEIDMAN, E. S. *Deaths of Man*, 1973.

Originally interested in suicide, this author has extended his research to include all death-related behavior. His highly personal book contains a section on clinical thanatology based on his own experience, as well as extracts from talks with a dying patient and an analysis of Herman Melville's struggle with the problem of death, e.g., in *Moby Dick*.

SHNEIDMAN, E. S. *Death: Current Perspectives*, 1976.

This is another anthology with very well chosen contemporary writings. Shneidman's interstitial materials captivate the reader by the balance of emotionality and scholarship.

WRITINGS ON TERMINAL CARE

Most articles and books in the field of thanatology deal with death from a variety of aspects and often try to illuminate several disparate problems. It was probably because of this that Weisman (1975), writing a chapter on thanatology in a large textbook of psychiatry, presented his material in a clear-cut manner to serve as a basis for subdividing thanatology.

Much of what has been written about death—be it connected with psychology, sociology, philosophy or religion—is motivated by a desire to clarify and improve conditions for the dying individual. The wish to help dying persons is unquestionably a strong incentive to thanatological work in general and many writers implicitly assume that their findings and ideas are applicable to this. In many works that appear to be devoted entirely to theoretical thanatological problems one suddenly comes across observations or arguments that are directly relevant to and valuable for daily work at a dying person's bed-side. In the anthologies and basic works cited above, for instance, only a few chapters deal directly with care of the dying, but elsewhere in the volumes there are additional data, opinions or discussions that are pertinent to practical terminal care.

SURVEY OF WORK ON PSYCHOLOGICAL TERMINAL CARE

The works summarized here have been selected subjectively from a wide range. I have tried to concentrate on those that are directly relevant to the special method for psychological terminal care described in this book. Works that consider psychological aspects of clinical thanatology fairly generally are presented first, followed by a review of writings where clinical thanatology is illustrated by means of a detailed description of one or occasionally a few dying patients.

General Works

EISSLER, K. *The Psychiatrist and the Dying Patient*, 1955.

This book, which has already been mentioned among the basic works on death, contains a great deal on thanatological theory and touches on philosophy and fiction. The author's aim is to show that the psychiatrist has a justifiable place in care of the dying, though he adds that to the best of his knowledge no one has ever questioned this. Note that the book was written in 1955.

Eissler gives penetrating descriptions of three cancer patients whom he followed as a psychiatrist while they were dying. Much of his clinical advice and opinions were new at the time and proved fruitful for clinical thanatology. It should be emphasized that, while Eissler is a psychoanalyst, it is clear that his treatment of these three patients is not psychoanalysis but a contact, tailored to meet the particular situation and referred to by him as psychotherapy. On the other hand, his insight into and interpretation of the patient's problems and his description of how best to support dying patients are formulated in a psychoanalytical frame.

It would be hard to summarize Eissler's line of thought and approach here but some of his central ideas should be mentioned. In contacts with dying patients, Eissler attributes great importance to what he terms "the gift situation." According to him, the psychiatrist must create the right opportunity at the right time to present the right "gift," which means that this must be done in a situation where the patient has a positive transference to the therapist and the gift acquires a symbolic significance for the patient. Consequently, the psychiatrist is required to understand the patient's needs better than he does himself. The gift must be made, moreover, before the need or wish has been verbalized and without expecting a gift in return.

These "gifts" are not primarily material so much as something one does unasked for the patient. One can give by trying to respond with imagination, perception and warmth to the needs that dying activates in the patient. Eissler mentions some fairly tangible gifts but mainly describes those of a psychological nature. He gives of his time and of himself. He even goes so far as to try to convey to the patient that a part of himself will die with the latter in order that they, in the patient's internal sphere, in a sense and to some extent, seem to die together.

The main emphasis in Eissler's work with the dying is on the importance and the manner in which the psychiatrist can support a patient's *individuality*. He formulates some pairs of opposites to characterize work with the dying:

> Warm, intimate feelings for the patient that do not amount to love (so-called sublimated love) in contrast to a reasonable distance with a matter-of-fact assessment of each step.

> The patient's conception of his own immortality and the psychiatrist's acceptance of this in contrast to behavior with the patient that is marked by the seriousness of the situation.

> The patient's anxiety while dying, an anxiety that the psychiatrist shares in a sense, in contrast to an awareness that

what is happening is an inevitable organic process that we all know has to occur.

The psychiatrist's despondency and feeling for the patient in contrast to grief and despair (e.g., on the part of relatives), which the psychiatrist must avoid.

Eissler refers to these four pairs of opposites as *paradoxes,* but, as a psychodynamic psychiatrist, he explains that instead of being peculiar to dying, they also occur in other contexts in a person's psychological life. He wants us to analyze and penetrate the paradoxes we encounter in the process of dying, understand them and realize that they are paradoxes not just for the patient but for us as well. He wants the psychiatrist to accept them, just as he accepts life's other paradoxes that are less anxiety-provoking for him.

Eissler also points out that, once a psychiatrist has built up a relationship with a dying patient, it is difficult, not to say impossible, for another psychiatrist to take it over either temporarily or permanently. The process of identification is extremely intense. Another point he makes is that a psychiatrist can be useful to the dying person in ways that relatives cannot on account of their love (or perhaps the opposite) for him and a preoccupation with grief, despair and other composite feelings.

RENNEKER, R. E. *Countertransference reactions to cancer,* 1957.

This article is based on psychological observations of what happened when several psychoanalysts undertook to give psychotherapy to women who had been treated for mammary cancer. It soon became clear that the therapists subconsciously hoped that this would effect a cure or prevent a recurrence. It is particularly noteworthy that when the disease showed signs of spreading or the patient began to die, the therapists reacted by withdrawing from the contact—they failed the patient. Countertransference became too strong.

ROSENTHAL, H. R. *Psychotherapy for the dying*, 1957.

The author wishes to draw attention to "a small segment of people with death fears which I should like to call the 'forgotten' patients—those who have been stricken by a fatal organic disease." The author attempts to systematize a psychotherapy for dying persons. The first task, in her view, is to determine whether the patient is aware, semi-aware or completely unaware that the disease is fatal. She shows that relatives and friends try to dispel anxiety and avoid discussing the disease. Consequently, the patient starts fearing his fear and this is one reason why it is necessary to have an independent therapist who is accustomed to handling anxiety with human warmth and psychological insight.

According to Rosenthal the following problems should be handled in the therapy:

guilt-feelings from various causes;

the feeling of not having had time for self-fulfillment;

loss of self-control;

the relationship between death and creativity.

These problems are illustrated with examples and the author briefly discusses how psychotherapy of dying persons differs from conventional psychotherapy, concluding that they have different goals but the same technique. She seems somewhat uncertain about this, however, and notes that it may be inadvisable to give a dying person analytical therapy. One must assess the patient's remaining ego-strength in relation to the strain of bringing up repressed, sensitive matters.

LESHAN, L. L. & GASSMAN, M. L. *Some observations of psychotherapy with patients suffering from neoplastic disease*, 1958.

LESHAN, L. L. & LESHAN, E., *Psychotherapy and the patient with a limited life span*, 1961.

The starting point here is whether cancer is a psychosomatic disease, i.e., the complex question of whether psychological factors can give rise to, elicit, be a contributory cause of or influence the course of a neoplastic disease. I find the conclusions rather unconvincing. In this context, however, LeShan devoted himself, alone or with various co-workers, to psychotherapy for dying persons. An assessment of his work with the dying is complicated by his interest in getting at the "psychosomatic" problem. LeShan's approach can be described as an intense psychotherapy with a psychoanalytical orientation and a substantial element of existential philosophy. It is not clear how many patients he treated, neither is one told what forms or stages of cancer they had.

There was a violent reaction when these articles appeared. It was thought almost offensive and obscene that a psychotherapist should devote himself to dying persons. This was more than five years after Eissler had written that no one could have any objection to psychiatric work with the dying. Attitudes seem to change; there have been conflicting reactions which have clearly been interpreted differently.

BARD, M.* *Implications of analytic psychotherapy with the physically ill,* 1959.

This author, who is a psychologist, belonged to a group which worked at the Memorial Hospital in New York on surveying and describing the emotional reactions of patients with various forms of cancer, i.e., their somatopsychic reactions in contrast to the psychosomatic problems considered by others. These studies have increased our knowledge and understanding of the psychological implications of cancer.

Bard takes up Renneker's observation that psychotherapists are unwilling to treat patients with a severe somatic disease, particularly if they are dying. He concludes with the hope that his views will stimulate psychotherapeutic work of this kind, pointing out that it is also personally rewarding and professionally satisfying. This is often overlooked.

---

* I should like to take this opportunity to thank Morton Bard, who was my first teacher on the psychological impact of cancer.

ARONSON, G. J. *Treatment of the dying person*, 1959.

This paper appeared in the anthology edited by Feifel. Aronson considers that the central task in contacts with the dying is to permit and help the patient to maintain as much as possible of the role which he finds important. Four rules are given by way of guidance:

> Never say anything to the patient that may elicit psychopathology.
>
> Never allow hope to die before the patient.
>
> Do not belittle the seriousness of the situation.
>
> Try to assess the time that remains for a satisfactory psychological functioning and make that time meaningful.

Aronson gives some clinical as well as more literary examples and then returns, like so many other writers, to Freud's assertion that we cannot imagine our own death, that we have a subconscious intimation of our own immortality. But if this is true, why do we still fear death? Aronson, who shares Freud's opinion, adds the pregnant comment that we want someone else to share our belief or confidence in our own immortality. In his opinion, a person who provides this support conveys a "gift" in Eissler's sense.

SAUNDERS, C. *Care of the Dying*, 1959.

This writer represents a completely different view of and solution to questions about care of the dying. Since 1959 Saunders has deliberately aimed at providing good terminal care by constructing an institution for the purpose. There are now several of these hospices in Great Britain and in the United States. The one created by Saunders, St. Christopher's Hospice in the south of London, seems to be the best in existence and can serve as a model here (Saunders, 1967, 1972). Its standard is that of an ordinary British hospital with the traditional hierarchy. Terminally ill patients are referred to it from other institutions and in addition to the hospitalized patients there are a great many outpatients. A clear policy has been developed in two respects. One concerns medication and nursing. The patients are well cared for, with the conscious aim of relieving all the discomforts and symptoms associated with dying. Saunders rightly claims that hospital care in general leaves much to be desired in this respect. The treatment of pain is a main issue (Twycross, 1978), but nausea, difficulty in breathing, insomnia, agitation and so on are all treated skillfully, sometimes unconventionally and always energetically (Saunders, 1976a, b). All the patients at St. Christopher's are terminally ill and no steps are taken to prolong life.

The other aspect to be emphasized is the spiritual or religious side of dying. The hospice follows a distinctly Christian line. This is evident from the fittings and decorations as well as from the number of clergymen and other representatives of various creeds one meets there. Dying and death are discussed openly if the patient so wishes and is able. It is said that no patient has a religious conviction forced upon him and this is no doubt true in a way. Yet the religious atmosphere is so pronounced that it is bound to make some impression. It seems hardly likely that dying patients, who tend to be lonely, questing, and charged with anxiety, would not be affected by seeing other patients, often a majority, assembled in prayer with the staff.

A well-known psychiatrist is attached to the hospice but is there only one day a week and, apart from research, devotes himself mainly to the staff and their psychological problems. He has published an assessment of St. Christopher's (Parkes, 1975). Medical and religious views on care of the dying at this institution have been gathered and discussed at length in various publications, but less interest seems to have been paid to psychological-psychiatric aspects (Craven & Wald, 1975; Liegner, 1975; Saunders, 1978).

Two developments of the hospice movement are, on the one hand, a growing tendency to care for dying persons at home as long as possible, and on the other, a tendency to place the unit itself in the middle of big general hospitals.

This applies for the Palliative Care Unit in Montreal (Mount, 1976), and the experience and work done in this unit are an important contribution. The patient can remain in the same hospital and one can avoid isolating or in a sense hiding the dying patient. Perhaps still more important is the impact on the care at other departments in the hospital where a palliative care unit is functioning. The excellent terminal care given at the unit of the Royal Victoria Hospital in Montreal has influenced care of the dying in the hospital as a whole in a profound way.

As the hospice movement and St. Christopher's have attracted a great deal of attention and are regarded by some as the ideal model for terminal care, I should like to say in conclusion that: the medical treatment, particularly the control of pain, is admirable; great efforts are made to create a warm, home-like setting that embraces the families and survivors as well as the dying patients; the strong emphasis on religion would be alien in practical hospital work in Sweden; and a hospital solely for dying persons, with all that this implies, could hardly be reconciled with the Swedish approach to care of the sick.

WEISMAN, A. D. & HACKETT, T. P. *Predilection to death: Death and dying as a psychiatric problem*, 1961.

Weisman is one of the pioneers of modern thanatology, besides being the central researcher and thinker on psychological care of the dying. He has conducted several important projects in clinical research, all dealing with dying and death. His design has been to pin down, describe and systematize knowledge about the nature of death in psychological, social and biological terms, to analyze the course of dying, describe the psychological processes in dying persons, formulate goals for work with the dying and also analyze why and in which ways hospital routines today are so unfamiliar with dying and death.

This article from 1961 contains the kernel of much that Weisman has subsequently extended and elaborated. He started with a special group of dying patients: persons who could predict that they would die in the near future, were able to talk openly about this, showed no anxiety or depression, appearing on the contrary contented that the end was at hand. Weisman termed this phenomenon "predilection to death." He analyzed five of these patients and was struck by the finding that people do exist who face their imminent death without anxiety or grief. It was from this experience that he extracted the foundation for his view of dying and his approach to the care of dying patients. (Patient no. 10 in my material exactly matches Weisman's "predilection to death.")

Since then he has developed his views and published a series of articles or books on related matters. An article from 1967 considers whether or not to tell the patient "the truth." In the same year he and Hackett published a detailed analysis of the concept of denial. In 1968 he and Kastenbaum, using the method known as "psychological autopsy," tried to identify and describe social and psychological signs of the preterminal and terminal phases in geriatric dying. In an extensive article from 1970, Weisman, instead of giving opinions and advice, described the unnecessary fears and misconceptions that circulate about psychiatric care of terminal patients.

The central work, *Dying and Denying,* which has been included above under basic works on thanatology, appeared in 1972 and was followed in 1974 by *The Realization of Death,* which is both a collected description of experiences from and a guide to the "psychological autopsy." This is now used not only after suicides but also for deaths in old age and for patients who die after a somatic disease. The latter book provides many clinical illustrations of the theoretical arguments in *Dying and Denying.* A well-known American textbook of psychiatry (1975) now includes a chapter by Weisman in which he presents a compressed account of his conceptual apparatus and attempts to systematize the material which in recent years has become the speciality known as thanatology.

Weisman's results are based on many years' experience of psychiatric work with dying patients. His activities and views have been constructed out of psychoanalytical insights and existentialist thinking (Weisman, 1965). Some of his central themes will be outlined here, particularly the aspects that are relevant for psychiatric work with the dying.

The concept of *psychosocial death* runs right through Weisman's work. He analyzes it, demonstrates how psychological and social factors on every level are interwoven, mark and sometimes determine how the individual perceives the process of dying and the meaning of death. He has followed, studied and compared persons who die in cancer, myocardial infarction or old age. His reports are strewn with specific observations that any doctor with a feeling for this aspect of life will recognize and be able to benefit from.

People die and death itself has a biological side, which is so tangible and has been studied in detail for so long in a biological framework that it dominates the scene and seems to be all-important. Weisman demonstrates that the psychological and social side of death is at least as significant. Besides determining how a person feels when faced with his own or a relative's death, psychosocial factors actually contribute to the when, where and how of an individual's death. These factors may be instrumental in bringing about death earlier or later than would have been the case if the psychosocial constellation had been different. People's lives are shortened or lengthened consciously or subconsciously by the fabric of psychosocial factors and biological events. A person's situation, the reactions of others, the attitudes of doctors and the workings of a hospital milieu all combine in such a way that death sometimes comes earlier than it might and is sometimes prolonged unnecessarily from the individual's point of view.

Death accordingly results from a number of interrelated social, psychological and biological factors and does not depend on just one of these. People do not die *of* cancer or a cardiac infarction. They may have these and other diseases, be very ill as a result and make a complete recovery or remain an invalid for many years. At a certain point, however, the medical, psychological and social constellation is such that they start dying and die. There are, moreover, ways of dying that have nothing to do with disease. One is suicide, where the psychosocial aspects obviously predominate.

It is the psychosocial nature of death that enables the rest of us—relatives, hospital staff, friends or religious companions— to come to the aid of the dying person, participate individually in the process of dying and help the patient.

Weisman draws attention to a number of *dimensions in our concept of death*:

> *impersonal death,* e.g., the significance of the dead body for a pathologist, or death as a statistic;
>
> *interpersonal death,* what one person's dying and death signifies for someone else;
>
> *intrapersonal death,* my own death.

It is intrapersonal death that elicits our anxiety for dying and death. Weisman analyzes these dimensions, with many clinical examples as well as valuable theoretical and practical reflections.

Another phenomenon that Weisman has considered at length is *denial* in connection with dying and death (1972; Weisman & Hackett, 1967). The term denial has been used for a long time by psychiatrists with a psychodynamic bent, as well as by somatic doctors and even laymen, though rather indiscriminately and in medical situations mostly when the opinions of patient and doctor differ.

In psychoanalytical terminology, denial was used originally as a label for a defense mechanism against threatening situations, actions and words. Reacting against the idea of denial as a mechanism that is triggered in specific situations, Weisman reformulates the term so that it becomes applicable in severe diseases and in the process of dying, thereby giving it a far more vital meaning. Weisman's denial is a total process of responding within a specific psychosocial context and he distinguishes between the "fact of denial" and the "process of denying." This process comprises several steps and ends in the fact of denial, the extent of which varies. The content of the steps in denying is determined by the psychosocial context, chiefly the relationship to and interaction with the person in front of whom one denies (cf. the interpersonal dimension of death). The external psychosocial factors likewise determine where, how and when the process of denying takes place and leads up to the result that others observe and call denial. The forms that denial takes during dying are influenced very considerably by relatives, doctors and other hospital staff. The dying person resorts to denial not simply to avoid a danger but to prevent the loss of significant relationships.

Denial obviously differs in degree and is seldom constant. Weisman provides a serviceable clinical classification: First-order denial concerns the primary facts of illness, second-order denial the extensions and implications of the illness, and third-order denial is a denial of death. The clinician should try to analyze the degree of denial that is present in the individual case and the psychological or somatic events that cause it to change.

Weisman also emphasizes and exemplifies a reality of far-reaching significance that has been neglected for a long time. It is meaningless to regard denial as an isolated attitude of the patient to his situation. One cannot understand it without recognizing the existence of its opposite, acceptance. These two are extremes on a very broad continuum. If a patient denies certain experiences, facts, etc., one should automatically assess what and how much he accepts, and only then consider how to go on communicating. A patient's awareness of a situation or certain aspects of this tends to lie between total denial and total acceptance; further it is not static. Weisman refers to this as having "middle knowledge." We are liable to be disdainful or irritated when patients and dying persons display "middle knowledge" about some part of what they are going through. We should instead analyze what the patient denies, what he accepts, and which middle way he adopts in relation to his doctor, his wife and others. This would increase our chances of sharing and easing his situation in ways that are psychologically meaningful for him.

Another psychoanalytical term with a specific meaning that Weisman redefines for use in the process of dying is *regression*. This he sees as a total phenomenon acting on many levels. It is more than a psychodynamic term. Regression is a form for existence and lies at the opposite end of a continuum from restitution. A regression of human existence has three aspects:

biodynamic regression, which is the psychological and behavioral counterpart of organic disease;

sociodynamic regression, a process that on various levels reduces and restricts a person's total social life;

psychodynamic regression, the counterpart of the psychiatric term expanded to include the existential dimension, which psychiatry seldom considers.

It is difficult to identify regression in the individual dying patient, but it is clear what is meant by the picture which Weisman gives on the basis of many years' experience.

In the two more recent books (1972, 1974), Weisman deals with the difficulty of registering and conveying what happens with sick and dying persons. What is essential may be missed in a description that covers a great many patients, while many sessions with a few patients may give a picture that is incomplete and onesided. Scientific ambition involves a risk of losing the heart of the matter one is trying to understand and formulate—the human and personal aspect of a situation. Descriptions of dying seem to oscillate between subjective, special observations and platitudinous generalizations. Weisman aims at an "intermediate generality" between the personal and the general.

Defense mechanisms borrowed from psychoanalytical theory are rejected by Weisman as a model for explaining the different ways in which people master difficult problems, particularly as he wishes to register a continuous event. Instead, he opts for a description of a person's "vulnerability," a term based on his own observations and experience and formulated in a set of poles between which moods, attitudes and behavior fluctuate during the course of dying. Seen from one angle, they express the dying person's vulnerability and from another the way in which he copes with the difficulties (1976a).

Weisman has constructed rating scales which yield numerical

values for an "index of vulnerability" and a "general coping strategy." The ratings can be repeated during the course of the process and express the difficulties encountered by dying persons and the ways in which one might be able to help them cope. Weisman has used this instrument with dying persons and suicide patients, to track down factors that determine vulnerability, indicate groups at risk and point to the need for psychosocial support (1976b).

Thanatological terminology has benefited greatly from Weisman's efforts to name many situations or factors that feature in the process of dying and in our view of death.

Dying and death are closely connected but differ conceptually. Weisman proposes that we refer to dying as terminality, which would comprise all the events, actions and processes that lead to organic death. Physically, dying is an absence of almost all healthy functions and the moment of death is when they all cease. Psychosocially, the meanings of dying and death are more personal.

Other terms suggested by Weisman are *"significant survival"* and *"purposeful death."* To quote Weisman, "Significant survival is a quality of life that means more than simply not to die. Purposeful death also means more than dying; it includes a measure of fulfillment, quiescence, resolution and even traces of personal development" (1972, p. 33-34). Weisman wishes us to realize that "unspecified emotional factors are significant determinants of the disposition to die." Patients are encountered who die "with yearning, acceptance, certainty, serenity and even a measure of impatience." Because these patients are willing to die without any signs of denial and anxiety, Weisman, as mentioned earlier, terms this *"predilection to death."*

The term that has attracted most attention and discussion is *"appropriate death."* This is an attempt to summarize the components of "a good death," i.e., the goal of psychological work with dying persons. Consequently, it also affords a contrast to our conventional conception of death as invariably associated with defeat, humiliation and the like. To quote Weisman again, "appropriate death is a form of purposeful death, but not every instance of purposeful death is an appropriate death" (1972, p. 37).

The definition which Weisman (1961) gives of appropriate

death runs as follows: "1) conflict is reduced; 2) compatibility with the ego ideal is achieved; 3) continuity of important relationships is preserved or restored; 4) consummation of a wish is brought about" (Weisman & Hackett, 1961, p. 248). Weisman expresses these ideas in various ways and emphasizes that this is an attempt to formulate an ideal. To illustrate his definition, he gives specific, practical examples that all serve to clarify the goal for psychological work with dying persons.

The dying person must be kept as free from pain and suffering as possible and one should do everything to prevent him becoming socially or emotionally isolated or impoverished. He should be allowed to function on as high a level as possible in the current situation. Conflicts should be brought up and if possible resolved, wishes satisfied if his condition permits in accordance with his ego ideal. He should be free to choose whom to have close, whom to relinquish, and to whom he firmly wishes to yield control of himself.

Summing up his definition, Weisman writes, "In short, an appropriate death is one which a person might choose for himself had he an option" (Inter. J. Psychiat. 2:191, 1966). This ". . . had he an option" points to an ideal for psychological work with dying persons and seems to be the key to what Weisman is driving at. Knowledge and human warmth are required to give a dying person an appropriate death. Weisman has few equals in his efforts to ensure that thanatologists and others at least have a goal to strive for.

ALDRICH, C. K. *The dying patient's grief*, 1963. *Some dynamics of anticipatory grief*, 1974.

The first, brief article concentrates mainly on the concept of *"anticipatory grief."* Anxiety about death is comprehensible to everyone and works on the subject are legion. Aldrich argues that another affect, grief, is equally important. The grief of a dying person is a reaction to loss of family members and relatives, parts of the body or its functions, aims in life and professional ambitions, etc., ultimately ending in grief for the imminent, final loss—of life itself. A patient who grieves or perhaps becomes depressed is reacting before the event, hence the term anticipatory grief. Many writers have described this feeling in dying persons as well as their relatives.

Aldrich also notes the similarity between the anticipatory grief of the dying person and that of relatives, though the latter also experience grief in the conventional sense after the patient's death. In the more recent work, he emphasizes the differences in dynamics. Grief in the accustomed sense is considered to diminish with time, whereas the anticipatory grief of both parties is assumed to increase as death approaches. In practice this is often not the case. For both parties the situation is no doubt modified by the balance between denial and acceptance (cf. p. 236), just as the ambivalence of interpersonal relationships no doubt influences anticipatory grief and the grief of relatives in different ways.

In a paper that appeared some years ago (Fulton & Fulton, 1971) anticipatory grief was discussed from various aspects and it was pointed out that patient and relatives both feel grief but have many other, frequently ambivalent feelings concurrently that color and modify this grief. Here, perhaps, is one of the reasons why relatives have difficulty in giving a dying person emotional help and support, a circumstance that both Eissler (1955) and Rosenthal (1957) have noted and which is one of the factors behind the design of my approach.

In the first article, Aldrich also takes up the question of a patient's strength of personality. Hospital staff frequently refer to and are impressed by a patient's strength and an apparent absence of this may be met with some disdain. Yet people who "appear strong" are liable to be misunderstood. There are persons with an ability to form warm, human relationships, many friends, perhaps a confident hope about a life hereafter, and an apparent adaptability to the symptoms of their disease. But loss and grief may often be more difficult to bear for them than for many other personalities; it is just their strength that enables them to hide their feelings from others. Persons who appear to accept death are quite often in a state of depression and what appears to be realistic courage is, in fact, a sign that they have given up and, if anything, welcome death.

Aldrich concludes with an important comment on whether or not to tell "the truth." Aldrich considers that right from the start of a contact one must let the patient choose between denial and acceptance. We must talk and behave in such a way that during the course of dying he is able to fluctuate between these two poles in the manner that suits him best in each situation.

HINTON, J. M. *The physical and mental distress of the dying,* 1963.

Several works on death, based on his own studies, have been presented by this writer, who is a professor of psychiatry in London. Surprising though it may seem, this article from 1963 was the first serious attempt by anyone to analyze and systematize the physical and psychological symptomatology of dying persons. It reports the number who are distressed, in what way, how different kinds of distress relate to the disease or personal life, and finally whether the distress changes as the patient approaches death. The study covers 102 patients who were expected to die within six months. With each one of them, Hinton had a 30-minute talk once a week until they died and also undertook a corresponding study on a control group of patients from the same hospital with relatively benign complaints. There is no room here to consider all the interesting and extensive data, but it can be noted that depression was found to be very common among the dying, an incidence of 45 percent compared with 37 percent for anxiety. The study is particularly valuable in that it goes beyond momentary observations and follows patients throughout the course of dying.

Hinton has also described attitudes to death among dying patients, including an analysis of whether one should or should not inform patients that they have a fatal disease and how they react to such a message (1966). Furthermore, he has presented a brief, clear and readable account of how he considers one should talk with dying persons (1967).

In a preliminary report on whether and in what way husband and wife can communicate when one of them is threatened by a fatal disease, Hinton (1970) notes that one-third of the dying were capable of talking realistically—though often for only a short time—about these questions with their partner.

In another paper (1971), he summarizes the difficulties of reporting in a scientific manner desires and views of patients during the course of dying. It can be hard to distinguish between the emotions and real needs of the dying person, and the observer is always involved in some way. One must always have a clear idea of why, how, when and by whom the problem is to be studied. Unless one does this, analyzes what is relevant to investigate and is aware of the investigation's own position, the result will be a series of false conclusions and distorted pictures of the quality of terminal care. This is an aspect that I, too, have tried to publicize on several occasions (Feigenberg, 1975a, Feigenberg & Fulton, 1976b) in Sweden.

There is a brief article by Hinton (1972) about conventional psychiatric consultations with 50 dying cancer patients at an oncologic clinic. In his studies of dying persons, Hinton (1975) has considered the extent to which the pre-morbid personality influences the reactions of cancer patients when they are dying. He studied 60 married patients who were terminally ill in cancer and tried to correlate various features of their pre-morbid personality with behavior during the disease. For this purpose he interviewed the husband/wife, the patient and the nurse. Hinton simply presents his observations and is well aware of the weaknesses of such a method.

The results support the view that the way a patient lives influences his manner of dying. It is noteworthy that no significant difference was found, in the degree of depression or anxiety when dying, between previously stable and neurotic persons. Difficulty in adapting to situations during life was associated with more rejection and reserve while dying, leading to loneliness and isolation. Adjustment difficulties earlier also gave a stronger tendency to depression and anxiety. Active persons with an ability to reach decisions displayed a greater awareness that they were dying, besides being more appreciative of the care they received. The ability to adapt to dying correlated clearly with a feeling of satisfaction with life, e.g., the experience of a happy marriage. The strength of religious belief had no effect on reactions in the face of death. While these and other findings may be debatable, it should be noted that the study has a simple design and demonstrates that these questions, about which so little is known, can be investigated in a manner that is meaningful even for the dying person.

GLASER, B. G. & STRAUSS, A. L. *Awareness of Dying,* 1965. *Time for Dying,* 1968.

These books, by two sociologists, report extensive studies on conditions for dying patients at a group of hospitals on the West Coast of the United States. Thanks to the design and presentation of this sociological research, the findings are of great value for persons engaged in care of the dying. The authors have developed a special sociological theory as a starting point and foundation for their research (1967). Their structure of problems around central themes produces a meaningful picture. Many details which one has noticed or wondered about in connection with care of the dying are integrated into an intelligible general pattern.

The central theme in the first of these two books is the *"awareness context,"* i.e., "what each interacting person knows of the patient's defined status, along with his recognition of the others' awarenesses of his own definition." Four types of awareness context are distinguished:

Closed awareness: The patient does not recognize his impending death even though the hospital personnel have the information.

Suspicion awareness: The patient does not know, but only suspects with varying degrees of certainty, that the hospital personnel believe him to be dying.

Mutual pretence: The patient and staff both know that the patient is dying but pretend otherwise.

Open awareness: Both staff and patient know that he is dying, and acknowledge it in their actions.

These four types of situations leave their mark on the interaction of the patient and his surroundings, bring out different attitudes in others and involve different risks. The authors analyze both the causes and the effects of transitions from one awareness context to another.

The second book describes the "trajectory of dying" that is common to all patients, though its duration and shape are often only vaguely perceived. There is an account of "critical junctures along the trajectory"; these, too, are usually overlooked or misunderstood. The trajectory may be rapid or slow and the former case may end in a sudden death that is expected or unexpected. A person whose death is sudden and unexpected may, in turn, have been aware or completely unaware that he would soon die. Similar distinctions can be made in a number of constellations involving varying degrees of awareness on the part of the dying person and those around him.

These books are not directly concerned with psychology but they nevertheless contain descriptions of situations, processes, conflicts and so on that constantly occur in work with the dying and have far-reaching psychological consequences.

During their studies these researchers were struck by the lack of a clear allocation of responsibility among the categories of staff when it came to reporting events and measures taken during the terminal phase. This applied not only to nurses (Quint, 1967), but also to other groups (Strauss et al., 1964). More than a decade later, a discussion has at last started on this subject—the lack of rules and regulations, aims and standards for terminal care (Kastenbaum, 1975b).

PATTISON, E. M. *The experience of dying,* 1967.

The thesis here, which I find debatable, is that anyone who is dying experiences certain universal emotions that are independent of culture, social order, belief or experience and that we meet these feelings each time we encounter a dying person.

The article is of interest because Pattison regards death and dying as a crisis. A crisis for Pattison seems to be a situation which a person feels that he does not have the resources to cope with. This generates anxiety, which prevents him from handling the situation. Pattison regards dying as such a situation and concludes that we have a chance of intervening. Although we cannot overcome the ultimate problem, death, we can at least help the dying person to tackle sub-aspects of the crisis that is inherent in the process of dying.

It seems to me that Pattison's description of experiences associated with dying do not require the use of the crisis concept. Helping dying persons to handle sub-problems does not necessarily amount to crisis intervention.

Pattison (1974a), like Weisman, has written a chapter on terminal care in an American textbook of psychiatry. This is an indication that psychological-psychiatric views on dying are at last attracting attention and being incorporated in psychiatry.

KUBLER-ROSS, E. *On Death and Dying,* 1969.

The strength of this world-famous book lies in the extracts from talks with dying persons. These show convincingly and very appealingly that dying persons want to talk, that one can talk with them and, finally, that such talks are meaningful and rewarding for both parties.

The book undoubtedly has an emotional appeal and its appearance coincided with the new wave of engaged interest in the problem of death. Yet the volume of work on terminal care was already very large, with descriptions of many different approaches, and many other writers (e.g., Weisman) had published case histories and accounts of their therapeutic contacts. Perhaps the much greater impact of this book by Kübler-Ross has to do with the self-recognition we experience on reading genuine, verbatim talks, particularly when dying persons talk about themselves. This response causes us to listen with particular attention.

The book also contains theoretical sections, of which the best-known concerns the division of dying into five stages: denial, anger, bargaining, depression and, finally, acceptance. This division into stages has been discussed on p. 138.

Kübler-Ross has been asked many questions in the course of her worldwide series of lectures and in 1974 she published some of her answers, which are brief and unequivocal. In this book, which is flat compared to her first one, she acknowledges that the work with dying patients has made her religious.

In a more recent book which she has contributed to and edited, Kübler-Ross (1975) clearly departs from her previous line of thought and presents dying as a period of growth and maturity. Death is seen as that which gives meaning to life. She emphasizes that death is nothing to be afraid of because she knows that it represents the gateway to a new existence. In addition to religious belief, her thoughts now include a touch of mysticism.

SHNEIDMAN, E. S. *Deaths of Man*, 1973.

Shneidman is, to the best of my knowledge, the first professor of thanatology and perhaps the first to define clinical thanatology as a special branch of thanatology. His experience of suicide patients and of dying persons and those they leave behind has prompted him to introduce the term "postvention" to complement prevention and intervention.

Shneidman also returns to his earlier work of creating a coherent system out of all death-related behavior (1963). The present book opens with verbatim texts of talks with a dying patient whom he managed and who agreed to have these talks recorded on videotape. Shneidman then uses this case as a starting point for clinical as well as theoretical arguments.

Two of Shneidman's characteristics are clear from this book, which actually contains a great deal of what he has written earlier elsewhere. The first is his involvement and willingness to talk emotionally about emotional reactions, his own as well as those of others. The second characteristic is that, like Weisman, he has done much to systematize thanatology and create its terminology.

Shneidman in recent years has devoted much energy to psychological care of the dying. His viewpoints in his anthology (1976) and an article in another anthology (1978) give a stimulating picture of ongoing thinking and creative development.

CASSEM, N. H. & STEWART, R. S. *Management and care of the dying patient,* 1975.

In the space of ten pages these authors achieve an admirable survey of problems in terminal care—including psychodynamic theory as well as clinical practice—without losing sight of the human aspects.

Recently Cassem (1978) has also contributed with a more extensive and informative chapter about care for the dying in a new textbook of psychiatry.

HAGGLUND, T-B. *Dying,* 1976.

The author describes several psychotherapies with dying persons (a child, a boy of 12 and several adults). Out of these experiences, plus a study of the famous Finish poetess Edith Södergran's poems, which are colored by the threat of death, he composes a picture of the psychology of dying and grief based on psychoanalytical theory. Defensive and creative processes constitute the central theme.

Case Reports

Therapists' descriptions of contacts with dying individuals make instructive and fascinating reading. They convey aspects of psychological terminal care which have no place in general, abstract reports. And when, as in the case of Eissler (1955), an author combines descriptions of individual patients with a discussion of his general approach to care of the dying, we are often in a better position to understand his method and attitudes.

The descriptions of individual patients in the publications mentioned below prompt another comment. Most of these authors work in the psychoanalytical frame of reference and employ its nomenclature. What they write, however, gives one the impression of a highly personal, subjective manner of supporting a dying person on the psychological plane. They make their own departures from psychoanalysis or psychotherapy, adapting their techniques to the situation at hand. It seems to be the individual therapist's own reaction to the meeting with a dying person that determines how he modifies or completely abandons the dicta of his training. The frequency of sessions and their length, the interpretations and active manipulation of the patient or the surroundings—all are utilized in a way that is foreign to classic psychoanalysis or psychotherapy in the psychoanalytical manner.

The book by Eissler (1955) referred to above centers on personal descriptions of three patients; these are most instructive and clearly indicate how Eissler departs from conventional psychoanalysis. It can be added that Eissler did not, in fact, follow any of these three patients right to the end.

Sandford published an article in 1952 about a very interesting case of a male patient with an obsessive-compulsive neurosis whom he treated psychoanalytically for four years. Later, when the patient got cancer of the lungs, the therapy was resumed and this part of the contact has been described, too (1957). Here, then, is a psychiatric case where, because the writer was already thoroughly acquainted with the patient, we get a unique insight into such a personality's perception of and reaction to death.

Saul (1959) describes his contact with a patient who was a doctor and had a more or less normal psyche. An account is given of this patient's psychological reactions during the last six months of his life, when he was aware that his cancer of the stomach would prove fatal.

Young (1960) writes about a woman of 51 to whom he gave psychotherapy but whose presenting symptoms were such that it was very difficult to determine whether their background was organic or psychological. She had suddenly fallen down as though dead, being unable to move or speak. The symptom disappeared but returned after a while. There was strong death-anxiety but this was complicated by ambivalent death-wishes. The problem of death was accentuated when a brother died and she also learned that her husband's severe hypertension would soon leave her a widow. During the first phase of the psychotherapy, she consulted several doctors in search of an organic explanation for the symptoms. All examinations were negative. In time her psychic condition improved and in analysis she achieved some insight into her relationship with the problem of death.

In this phase it was found that she had a cancer of the skin, followed shortly afterwards by esophageal cancer. The psychotherapy was continued until she died about a year later. After the therapist had been summoned to his father's death-bed in the middle of a session with the patient, they were able to work on their conscious and subconscious feelings about death. The patient's strength ebbed rapidly but she still greatly needed the analyst's help to work through childhood and other experiences that had a bearing on her death-anxiety and other psychological symptoms. After her death the husband, who was still alive, certified that throughout the course of her disease she had benefited greatly from her relationship with the psychoanalyst.

Joseph (1962) describes her contact with a woman of 27 whom she had given psychoanalysis for an anxiety neurosis. The therapy proved successful and they were discussing its conclusion when it was found that the young woman had an inoperable cancer of the colon with metastases in the liver, making it obvious that she had very little time left. This radically changed the therapist's role and the content of the therapy. She became important for the patient in quite another way and many emotions were aroused in her by this experience of a young woman's dying and death.

Transference and countertransference are described at length and movingly, not as theoretical concepts but through a vivid description of both parties' feelings, thoughts and behavior. Joseph encountered overwhelming problems during the course of the contact and found some of the answers in Eissler's (1955) book, an experience which she shares with many others who work with the dying.

Norton (1963) gives a detailed account of her treatment of a 32-year-old mother with two children during the last three months of her life. The patient was a warm, intelligent and talented woman who at the end of her second pregnancy (cf. patient B) was found to have a carcinoma of the breast, which greatly influenced her feelings for this second son. Her family and friends shrank from the task of supporting this patient and the author acquired an increasingly important place in her existence. A very instructive case history is presented and discussed with Eissler's ideas (1955) in mind. The writer describes how the patient tested her at first and gives a detailed account of her own experiences during the contact with this dying person.

Roose (1969a, b) is a psychoanalyst who has been attached for a long time to a psychiatric liaison service at a large teaching hospital in New York. One of his tasks is to act as a psychiatrist when psychological problems arise in the medical care.

Roose gives a detailed account of his contact with a patient with a deviant personality, who was dying of cancer of the lungs and announced at the start that he would commit suicide if his disease turned out to be cancer. Roose also illustrates experiences of the therapist and shows that with a patient who is dying, transference can serve as a therapeutic instrument rather than being used to interpret psychological mechanisms. Similarly, he tries to clarify his own countertransference to this dying man. The second of these two articles contains a more general discussion of psychological problems and what the psychiatrist can do for dying persons.

Strauss and Glaser (1970) are two sociologists whose research has been discussed above (p. 243). In this analysis of what happens in the care of a single patient, they illustrate the two concepts which they introduce: death trajectory and awareness context. The patient in question is a "difficult" woman. What happens up to her death is described from various angles, e.g., by two nurses, one of whom was actively responsible for the patient's care, whereas the other observed the events for a scientific report. The authors give many clear illustrations of their theories and conclude with a discussion of the relationship between theories based on sociological studies of large materials, such as their earlier works (1965, 1968), and experience from a single case.

Levine (1972) and *Trombley* (1972), both psychiatrists, relate their feelings and thoughts after learning that they had leukemia. They both deal with reactions to disease and death, their thoughts about family, colleagues and patients. Maurice Levine, who was a professor and the prominent head of a large psychiatric clinic, had for many years distributed occasional circulars to his staff, "Memos from ML." This is the last one, written a month before he died. Trombley wrote his essay in May 1967 and died two months later.

Leigh (1974) describes a psychotherapeutic contact with a woman of 35 who had attempted suicide when she had a very advanced mammary cancer with metastases. The contact started at the hospital immediately after the suicidal attempt, continued on an outpatient basis and was maintained by telephone up to the end as the patient became very weak and was cared for at home. Leigh considers that with such a dying patient the psychiatrist should maintain a psychotherapeutic relationship but at the same time keep in touch with the family and the somatic doctors. I have difficulty in seeing how these two aspects can be combined.

Muslin et al. (1974) describe two patients of the same age with carcinoma of the lung, both with a low social status, one white, the other black and with quite different personalities. The two established a friendship and the author, a psychiatrist, looked after them both. As their needs in this situation were very different, to help them he had to be the idealized, omnipotent and magical doctor for one and an admired, loving parent for the other. He showed how, as a doctor with a psychodynamic insight into the patient's psyche, one must enter with empathy into the needs of the dying person. One of these patients, who had been excluded from human companionship for years, summarized his experience of the support he had received in the words, "I had to catch cancer to join society."

Lines of Development

It may be asked whether one can detect a development in the psychological treatment of dying patients during the period in which contemporary psychological-psychiatric knowledge has been applied to care of the dying. This period amounts to approximately two decades and it is obvious that matters have developed. There are the achievements of the authors mentioned above and many others, besides which they have influenced one another in various ways and stimulated each other's research. Many have arranged to cooperate, combined in scientific organizations or in the joint publication of journals with a thanatological line. It would nevertheless seem very difficult to attempt to write a "history" of the brief period that has passed. Quite recently, however, such an attempt has in fact been made.

Levinson (1975) distinguishes three phases in works on the dying and terminal care. The first opens with Eissler's book in 1955 and includes the works mentioned above on solitary patients by Saul (1959), Young (1960), Norton (1963) and Roose (1969a). In this period, according to the author, individual psychotherapy and, quite frequently, analysis were provided for young, intelligent, cultivated, mature persons who had adjusted to reality. The second phase is marked by Kübler-Ross's (1969) book and during this period one was mainly concerned, according to Levinson, with religious middle-class patients, responsible, hardworking, self-sacrificing, family-oriented, with roots in established society. The third phase is represented by several authors who have published general surveys rather than clinical material, the examples given including Feifel (1959b), Brim et al. (1970) and Kastenbaum and Aisenberg (1972).

While there is some truth in this description, a picture of the development of terminal care based solely on this literature is bound to be biased. There is no mention at all of writers such as Weisman, the team around Saunders or the work of Hinton. The psychological quality of terminal care has undoubtedly been poor and remains so on the whole. Still, there are many who have done all they can for people in this situation in various parts of the world and this is not mentioned in Levinson's account, which appears to be confined to development in the United States. He concludes, moreover, that individuals with a marked psychopathology and low social status have not been considered or benefited from psychological terminal care during any of these periods. However, several reports (Duff & Hollingshead, 1968; Kosa et al., 1969) indicate that such patients in the United States have received very poor medical care, somatic as well as psychiatric, regardless of whether or not they were dying. Similarly, just as wealthy persons with useful contacts have obtained good medical service in general, so have they to some extent been able to "purchase" better terminal care than others.

Appendix II

Data on the Patients

Data on the 38 patients on whom this study is based are presented in tabular form below. The patients are listed in chronological sequence. The first one died in October 1968, the last in November 1975.

The reason for referral given here is an attempt to summarize the note of referral, not a direct quotation from this. The duration of my contact with a patient before starting the actual terminal care is given approximately in months.

In an attempt to indicate the structure of the terminal contact I have listed its duration in weeks, the number of talks and the approximate time in hours spent. This time comprises my direct talks with the patient and my talk with relatives at the beginning of the contact.

No.	Sex	Age at death	Diagnosis	Reason for referral	Contact before terminal care (months)	Terminal contact (weeks)	No. of talks	Total time spent (hours)
1	f	44	Hodgkin's disease	depression	9	8	3	3
2	f	47	Carcinoma of the breast	depression	6	8	2	2
3	f	43	Carcinoma of the breast	"attempted suicide" via cancer	6	24	11	7
4	m	59	Carcinoma of the lung	psychiatric contact desired by relatives	0	16	19	10.5
5	f	54	Carcinoma of the pancreas	need to relieve pain	5	4	9	6
6	f	34	Carcinoma of the colon	terminal care requested by patient	0	7	16	7
7 (patient A)	m	16	Osteogenic sarcoma	anxiety	0	9	25	10
8 (patient B)	f	26	Carcinoma of the colon	terminal care needed	0	5	12	6
9	f	50	Carcinoma of the breast	marital conflict	0.5	2	12	2.5
10	m	49	Carcinoma of the larynx	severe pains, problems with medication	0	2	2	1.5
11	f	40	Carcinoma of the cervix	depression	3	4	3	3
12	f	41	Carcinoma of the breast	psychiatric contact needed	6	12	7	5
13	f	44	Carcinoma of the ovary	anxiety	0	1	6	3.5

No.	Sex	Age at death	Diagnosis	Reason for referral	Contact before terminal care (months)	Terminal contact (weeks)	No. of talks	Total time spent (hours)
14	f	47	Carcinoma of the cervix	reaction to disclosure of diagnosis	3	12	7	5.5
15	f	40	Carcinoma of the ovary	appeal for euthanasia	0	1	6	3
16 (patient E)	f	60	Carcinoma of the breast	need for psychological support	20	12	8	5
17	f	65	Carcinoma of the lung	pains	3	4	12	5
18	f	37	Carcinoma of the ovary	anxiety	4	3	12	5
19	f	22	Carcinoma of the ovary	anxiety	0.5	3	10	5
20	f	25	Hypernephroma	terminal care needed	0	7	11	6
21	f	54	Carcinoma of the thyroid	depression	52	20	7	5
22	f	75	Carcinoma of the breast	depression	16	8	2	2
23 (patient D)	f	47	Malignant melanoma	requested contact with psychiatrist	0	17	18	14
24	f	37	Carcinoma of the rectum	tragic situation	4	16	13	6.5
25	f	40	Carcinoma of the breast	depression	32	10	10	4
26	f	42	Malignant melanoma	anxiety	10	9	14	5
27	m	58	Carcinoma of the testicle	depression	0	12	11	8.5

No.	Sex	Age at death	Diagnosis	Reason for referral	Contact before terminal care (months)	Terminal contact (weeks)	No. of talks	Total time spent (hours)
28 (patient C)	m	40	Carcinoma of the lung	death-anxiety	0	9	10	6
29	f	29	Carcinoma of the cervix	death-anxiety	3	12	18	8
30	f	47	Carcinoma of the ovary	appeal for euthanasia	0	4	21	15
31	f	28	Hodgkin's disease	psychiatric contact needed	3.5	12	12	10
32	f	23	Carcinoma of the cervix	suicidal thoughts and death-anxiety	3	56	34	20
33	f	51	Carcinoma of the ovary	anxiety	28	12	3	2
34	f	50	Carcinoma of the breast	applied herself for anxiety	8	20	21	13
35	m	67	Malignant melanoma	terminal care needed	7	28	6	4
36	f	60	Carcinoma of the breast	anxiety due to spread of tumor	24	20	5	5
37	f	53	Carcinoma of the cervix	death-anxiety	0	19	18	11
38	f	54	Carcinoma of the breast	anxiety about the disease	16	8	14	5.5

Appendix III

Criteria for Assessment of Terminal Care

This list of variables or items represents a preliminary attempt to specify and systematize the problems and questions that one would like to find answers to in a work on psychological terminal care. It would help to overcome the difficulties which, to some extent, are inherent in all clinical thanatology if reports or assessments of a method were designed to cover as many of these points as possible. This would also make comparisons easier. The scheme may also be used when reading thanatological works; in each case it may be constructive to ask oneself whether, to what extent and in what ways the problems listed here are illuminated and which conclusions can be drawn.

This suggested scheme has been developed, expanded and modified in the course of my work in this field and I hope that it will continue to be adapted and supplemented in the future.

1. *Target group for the care*
   patient
   relative
   personnel (e.g. supervision, group talks, "psychological autopsy")
   doctor
   nurse
   other personnel

2. *Characteristics of the patient(s)*
age
pre-morbid personality
level of intelligence
mental status
occupational and social status
family relations

3. *Where is the care given?*
at home
at an institution
   hospital
   nursing home
   institution for the dying (hospice, palliative care unit)
elsewhere

4. *Cause of dying*
illness
   diagnosis
   stage
   course
old age
accident
suicide
violence

5. *Who gives the care?*
doctor in somatic medicine
nurse
social worker
psychologist
psychiatrist
thanatologist
clergyman
relative
other

6. *Training and competence of caregiver in addition to occupational training*
psychology
psychotherapy
crisis intervention
spiritual care
thanatology

7. *Orientation and content of the terminal care*
psychological/psychiatric
    supportive and comforting
    promoting insight
    psychodynamic
    psychoanalytical
    client-centered psychotherapy (Rogers)
    behavioral therapy
    psychopharmacological
religious
philosophical
transcendental

8. *Structure of the contact*
number of contacts
frequency of contacts
total time spent
duration of each contact
changes in frequency and duration
setting for the contacts

9. *Aim of the terminal care*
care of the dying person
education and training
thanatological knowledge

10. *Methodological approach*
listen
establish a dialogue
interpret
share experiences and feelings

11. *Personality and attitudes of the therapist*

12. *Therapist's experience*
    emotional reactions
       grief
       depression
       anxiety
       aggressiveness
       feelings of guilt
    opportunities for unburdening
    need for supervision

13. *Evaluation*
    effects on
       the patient while dying
       relatives before and after the death
       personnel
       the public
       medical care
       the therapist
    insight and knowledge gained
    fields of application

14. *Comparison with other methods for terminal care*

References

ABRAMS, R. D. The patient with cancer—his changing pattern of communication. *New Engl. J. Med.*, 274:317-322, 1966.

ABRAMSON, R. A dying patient: The question of euthanasia. *Int. J. Psychiat. in Med.*, 6:431-454, 1975.

ALDRICH, C. K. The dying patient's grief. *JAMA*, 184:329-331, 1963.

ALDRICH, C. K. Some dynamics of anticipatory grief. In: B. Schoenberg, A. C. Carr, A. H. Kutscher, D. Peretz, and I. Goldberg (Eds.), *Anticipatory Grief*. New York: Columbia University Press, 1974, pp. 3-9.

ARIES, P. *Western Attitudes Toward Death: From the Middle Ages to the Present.* Baltimore: Johns Hopkins University Press, 1974, pp. 111.

ARONSON, G. J. Treatment of the dying person. In: H. Feifel (Ed.), *The Meaning of Death.* McGraw-Hill, 1959, pp. 251-258.

AUGUSTINE, M. J. & KALISH, R. A. Religion, transcendence, and appropriate death. *J. Transpersonal Psychol.*, 7:1-13, 1975.

BAIDER, A. L. *Family Structure and the Process of Dying: A Study of Cancer Patients and Their Family Interaction.* Boston: Dissertation, 1973.

BARD, M. Implications of analytic psychotherapy with the physically ill. *Amer. J. Psychother.*, 13:860-871, 1959.

BEIGLER, J. S. Anxiety as an aid in the prognostication of impending death. *Arch. Neurol. Psychiat.*, 77:171-177, 1957.

BERMANN, E. *Scapegoat. The Impact of Death-Fear on an American Family.* Ann Arbor: Univ. Michigan Press, 1973, p. 357.

BLEULER, M., WILLI, J., & BUHLER, H. R. Akute psychische Begleiterscheinungen körperlicher Krankheiten. "Akuter exogener Reaktions-Typus." *Ubersicht und neue Forschungen.* Stuttgart: Thieme Verl. 1966, p. 208 (in German).

BONHOEFFER, K. Die Psychosen im Gefolge von akuten Infektionen, Allgemeinerkrankungen und inneren Erkrankungen. In: G. Aschaffenburg, *Handbuch der Psychiatrie.* Spezieller Teil, 3 Abt. 1. Hälfte. pp. 1-118. Leipzig und Wien: F. Deuticke, 1912 (in German).

BORKENAU, F. The concept of death. *The Twentieth Century*, 157:313-329, 1955.

BRIM, O. G., JR., FREEMAN, H. E., LEVINE, S., & SCOTCH, N. A. (Eds.). *The Dying Patient.* New York: Russell Sage Foundation, 1970, p. 390.

BROMBERG, W. & SCHILDER, P. Death and dying: A comparative study of the attitudes and mental reactions toward death and dying. *Psychoanal. Rev.*, 20:133-185, 1933.

BROMBERG, W. & SCHILDER, P. The attitude of psychoneurotics towards death. *Psychoanal. Rev.*, 23:1-25, 1936.

263

264   Terminal Care

Bruhn, J. G., Paredes, A., Adsett, C. A., & Wolf, S. Psychological predictors of sudden death in myocardial infarction. *J. Psychosomat. Res.*, 18:187-191, 1974.

Burton, A. Attitudes toward death of scientific authorities on death. *Psychoanal. Rev.*, 65:415-432, 1978.

Campbell, P. Suicide among cancer patients. *Conn. Health Bull.*, 80:207-212, 1966.

Cassem, N. H. Treating the person confronting death. In: A. M. Nicholi, Jr. (Ed.), *The Harvard Guide to Modern Psychiatry.* Cambridge: Harvard University Press, 1978, pp. 579-606.

Cassem, N. H. & Stewart, R. S. Management and care of the dying patient. *Int. J. Psychiat. in Med.*, 6:293-304, 1975.

Chandler, K. A. Three processes of dying and their behavioral effects. *J. Consult. Psychol.*, 29:296-301, 1965.

Choron, J. *Death and Western Thought.* New York: Collier Books, 1963, p. 320.

Choron, J. *Death and Modern Man.* New York: Collier Books, 1964, p. 278.

Clark, J. J. & Levy, N. B. Reluctance to accept life-saving treatment. *Int. J. Psychiat. in Med.*, 6:561-569, 1975.

Cramond, W. A. Psychotherapy of the dying patient. *Br. Med. J.*, 3:389-393, 1970 (Aug. 15).

Crane, D. *The Sanctity of Social Life: Physicians' Treatment of Critically Ill Patients.* New York: Russell Sage Foundation, 1975, p. 285.

Craven, J. & Wald, F. S. Hospice care for dying patients. *Amer. J. Nursing,* 75:1816-1822, 1975.

Cullberg, J. *Kris och utveckling.* Stockholm: Natur & Kultur, 1975, p. 167 (in Swedish).

Danto, B. The cancer patient and suicide. *J. Thanat.*, 2:596-600, 1972.

Davies, R. K., Quinlan, D. M., McKegney, F. P., & Kimball, C. P. Organic factors and psychological adjustment in advanced cancer patients. *Psychosomat. Med.*, 35:464-471, 1973.

Dorpat, T. L., Anderson, W. F., & Ripley, H. S. The relationship of physical illness to suicide. In: H. L. P. Resnik (Ed.), *Suicidal Behaviors. Diagnosis and Management.* Boston: Little, Brown, 1968, pp. 209-219.

Duff, R. S. & Hollingshead, A. B. *Sickness and Society.* New York: Harper & Row, 1968, p. 390.

Eissler, K. R. (1955) *The Psychiatrist and the Dying Patient.* New York: International Universities Press, p. 338. Paperback, 1969.

Erikson, E. H. *Insight and Responsibility.* New York: Norton, 1964, p. 256.

Ettlinger, R. Evaluation of suicide prevention after attempted suicide. *Acta Psychiat. Scand. Suppl.*, 260, p. 135, 1975.

Farberow, N. & Shneidman, E. S. *The Cry for Help.* New York: McGraw-Hill, 1961, p. 398.

Farberow, N. L., Ganzler, S., Cutter, F., & Reynolds, D. An eight-year survey of hospital suicides. *Life-Threatening Behavior*, 1:184-202, 1971.

Feifel, H. Attitudes of mentally ill patients toward death. *J. Nerv. Ment. Dis.*, 122:375-380, 1955.

FEIFEL, H. Attitudes toward death in some normal and mentally ill populations. In: H. Feifel (Ed.), *The Meaning of Death*. New York: McGraw-Hill, 1959a, pp. 114-130.

FEIFEL, H. (Ed.). *The Meaning of Death*. New York: McGraw-Hill, 1959b, p. 351.

FEIFEL, H. Religious conviction and fear of death among the healthy and the terminally ill. *J. Sci. Study Religion*, 13:353-360, 1974.

FEIFEL, H. (Ed.). *New Meanings of Death*. New York: McGraw-Hill, 1977, p. 367.

FEIFEL, H., FREILICH, J., & HERMANN, L. J. Death fear in dying heart and cancer patients. *J. Psychosomatic Res.*, 17:161-166, 1973.

FEIFEL, H., HANSON, S., JONES, R., & EDWARDS, L. Physicians consider death. *Proc. 75th Ann. Convention Amer. Psychological Assn.*, 1967, pp. 201-202.

FEIFEL, H. & HELLER, J. Normalcy, illness, and death. *Proc. Third World Congress Psychiat.*, 2:1252-1256, 1961.

FEIFEL, H. & HERMANN, L. J. Fear of death in the mentally ill. *Psychol. Rep.*, 33:931-938, 1973.

FEIGENBERG, L. Döden och döendet. *Läkartidningen*, 68:5811-5821, 1971a (in Swedish).

FEIGENBERG, L. Människovärdig död. *Läkartidningen*, 68:5965-5975, 1971b (in Swedish).

FEIGENBERG, L. Läkaren och döden. *Läkartidningen*, 68:6103-6112, 1971c (in Swedish).

FEIGENBERG, L. Döden och dödsproblematiken. Tankar om döden i samhälle och sjukvård. *Läkartidningen*, 71:3766-3770, 1974 (in Swedish).

FEIGENBERG, L. Lättvindigt om terminalvård. *Läkartidningen*, 72:4850, 1975a (in Swedish).

FEIGENBERG, L. Care and understanding of the dying: A patient-centered approach. *Omega*, 6:81-94, 1975b.

FEIGENBERG, L. & FULTON, R. Döden i Sverige förr och nu. *Läkartidningen*, 73:2179-2182, 1976a (in Swedish).

FEIGENBERG, L. & FULTON, R. Vård av döende. *Läkartidningen*, 73:2253-2258, 1976b (in Swedish).

FEIGENBERG, L. & FULTON, R. Care of the dying: A Swedish perspective. *Omega*, 8:215-228, 1977.

FEIGENBERG, L. & SHNEIDMAN, E. S. Clinical thanatology and psychotherapy: Some reflections on caring for the dying person. *Omega*, 10:1-8, 1979.

FREUD, S. (1915) Thoughts for the times on war and death. *Standard Edition*. London: Hogarth Press, Vol. 14, pp. 273-302.

FREUD, S. (1920) Beyond the pleasure principle. *Standard Edition*. London: Hogarth Press, Vol. 18, pp. 57-143.

FROMM-REICHMANN, F. *Psychoanalysis and Psychotherapy. Selected Papers*. Chicago: University of Chicago Press, 1959, p. 350.

FULTON, R. (Ed.). *Death and Identity*. New York: Wiley & Sons, 1965, p. 415.

FULTON, R. (Ed.) in collaboration with BENDIKSEN, R. *Death and Identity*. Revised edition. Bowie, Md.: Charles Press, 1976, p. 448.

FULTON, R. (with the assistance of CARLSON, J., KROHN, K., MARKUSEN, E., & OWEN, G.) *Death, Grief and Bereavement: A Bibliography 1845-1975*. New York: Arno Press, 1977a.

FULTON, R. The sociology of death. *Death Education*, 1:15-25, 1977b.

FULTON, R. & FULTON, J. A psychosocial aspect of terminal care: Anticipatory grief. *Omega*, 2:91-100, 1971.

GIFFORD, S. Some psychoanalytic theories about death: A selective historical review. *Ann. N.Y. Acad. Sci.*, 164:638-668, 1969.

GLASER, B. G. Disclosure of terminal illness. *J. Health Hum. Behav.*, 7: 83-91, 1966.

GLASER, B. G. & STRAUSS, A. L. *Awareness of Dying*. Chicago: Aldine, 1965, p. 305.

GLASER, B. G. & STRAUSS, A. L. *The Discovery of Grounded Theory: Strategies for Qualitative Research*. Chicago: Aldine, 1967, p. 271.

GLASER, B. G. & STRAUSS, A. L. *Time for Dying*. Chicago: Aldine, 1968, p. 270.

GODIN, A. (Ed.). *Death and Presence. The Psychology of Death and the After-Life. Studies in the Psychology of Religion (V)*. Brussels: Lumen Vitae Press, 1972, p. 316.

GOLDBERG, I. K., MALITZ, S., & KUTSCHER, A. H. (Eds.). *Psychopharmacological Agents for the Terminally Ill and Bereaved*. New York: Columbia University Press, 1973, p. 339.

GREENSON, R. R. Empathy and its vicissitudes. *Int. J. Psycho-Anal.*, 41: 418-424, 1960.

HACKETT, T. P. & CASSEM, N. H. Patients facing sudden cardiac death. In: B. Schoenberg, A. C. Carr, D. Peretz, and A. H. Kutscher (Eds.), *Psychosocial Aspects of Terminal Care*. New York: Columbia University Press, 1972, pp. 47-56.

HACKETT, T. P. & WEISMAN, A. D. Denial as a factor in patients with heart disease and cancer. In: L. P. White (Ed.), *Care of Patients with Fatal Illness. Ann. N.Y. Acad Sci.*, 164:802-817, 1969.

HAGGLUND, T-B. *Dying. A Psychoanalytic Study with Special Reference to Individual Creativity and Defensive Organization*. New York: International Universities Press, 1978, p. 259.

HAMILTON, J. W. Some comments about Freud's conceptualization of the death instinct. *Int. Rev. Psycho-Anal.*, 3:151-164, 1976.

HICKS, W. & DANIELS, R. S. The dying patient, his physician and the psychiatric consultant. *Psychosomatics*, 9:47-52, 1968.

HINTON, J. The physical and mental distress of the dying. *Quart. J. Med.*, 32:1-21, 1963.

HINTON, J. Facing death. *J. Psychosomatic Res.*, 10:22-28, 1966.

HINTON, J. *Dying*. Penguin Books, 1967, p. 208.

HINTON, J. Communication between husband and wife in terminal cancer. Paper presented at the 2nd Inter. Conference on Social Science and Medicine in Aberdeen, Sept. 1970.

HINTON, J. Assessing the views of the dying. *Soc. Sci. and Med.*, 5:37-43, 1971.

HINTON, J. Psychiatric consultation in fatal illness. *Proc. Roy. Soc. Med.*, 65:1035-1038, 1972.

HINTON, J. The influence of previous personality on reactions to having terminal cancer. *Omega*, 6:95-111, 1975.

HOLT, H. Existential psychoanalysis. In: A. M. Freedman, H. I. Kaplan, and B. J. Sadock (Eds.), *Comprehensive Textbook of Psychiatry*, 2nd Edition, Vol. 1. Baltimore: Williams & Wilkins, 1975, pp. 661-668.

HOWARD, J. D. Fear of death. *J. Indiana St. Med. Ass.*, 54:1773-1779, 1961.

ISAACS, B., GUNN, J., MCKECHAN, A., MCMILLAN, I., & NEVILLE, Y. The concept of pre-death. *Lancet*, 1115-1119, May 29, 1971.

JANIS, I. L. A paradoxical effect of stress: Unrepression (Chap. 16). In: *Psychological Stress. Psychoanalytic and Behavioral Studies of Surgical Patients*. New York: John Wiley & Sons, 1958, pp. 179-194.

JOSEPH, F. Transference and countertransference in the case of a dying patient. *Psychoanal. Rev.*, 49:21-34, 1962.

KASTENBAUM, R. The reluctant therapist. *Geriatrics*, 18:296-301, 1963.

KASTENBAUM, R. The realm of death: An emerging area in psychological research. *J. Human Relations*, 13:538-552, 1965.

KASTENBAUM, R. On the future of death: Some images and options. *Omega*, 3:307-318, 1972.

KASTENBAUM, R. Is death a life crisis? On the confrontation with death in theory and practice: In: N. Datan & L. H. Ginsberg (Eds.), *Life-Span Developmental Psychology. Normative Life Crises*. New York: Academic Press, 1975a, pp. 19-50 .

KASTENBAUM, R. Toward standards of care for the terminally ill: That a need exists. *Omega*, 6:77-79, 1975b.

KASTENBAUM, R. Toward standards of care for the terminally ill. Part II: What standards exist today? *Omega*, 6:289-290, 1975c.

KASTENBAUM, R. Toward standards of care for the terminally ill. Part III: A few guiding principles. *Omega*, 7:191-193, 1976.

KASTENBAUM, R. & KASTENBAUM, B. S. Hope, survival, and the caring environment. In: E. Palmore and F. C. Jeffers (Eds.), *Prediction of Life Span*. Lexington, Mass.: Heath, 1971, pp. 249-271.

KASTENBAUM, R. & AISENBERG, R. *The Psychology of Death*. New York: Spinger, 1972, p. 498. Concise Edition, 1976, p. 446.

KATZ, R. L. *Empathy. Its Nature and Uses*. New York: Free Press of Glencoe, 1963, p. 210.

KAUFMANN, W. Existentialism and death. In: H. Feifel (Ed.), *The Meaning of Death*. New York: McGraw-Hill, 1959, pp. 39-63.

KOENIG, R. R. Fatal illness: A survey of social service needs. *Social Work*, 13:85-90, 1968.

KOENIG, R. R. Anticipating death from cancer—physician and patient attitudes. *Michigan Med.*, 68:899-905, 1969.

KOSA, J., ANTONOVSKY, A., & ZOLA, I. K. *Poverty and Health. A Sociological Analysis*. Cambridge, Mass.: Harvard University Press, 1969, p. 449.

KUBLER-ROSS, E. *On Death and Dying*. New York: Macmillan, 1969, p. 260.

KUBLER-ROSS, E. *Questions and Answers on Death and Dying*. New York: Collier Books, 1974, p. 177.

KUBLER-ROSS, E. *Death—the Final Stage of Growth*. Englewood Cliffs, N.J.: Prentice-Hall, 1975, p. 175.

LAPLANCHE, J. (1970) *Life and Death in Psychoanalysis*. Baltimore: Johns Hopkins University Press, 1976, p. 148.

LEIBER, L., PLUMB, M. M., GERSTENZANG, M. L., & HOLLAND, J. The communication of affection between cancer patients and their spouses. *Psychosom. Med.*, 38:379-389, 1976.

LEIGH, H. Psychotherapy of a suicidal, terminal cancer patient. *Int. J. Psychiat. in Med.*, 5:173-182, 1974.

LESHAN, L. L. & GASSMANN, M. L. Some observations on psychotherapy with patients suffering from neoplastic disease. *Amer. J. Psychother.*, 12:723-734, 1958.

LESHAN, L. L. & LESHAN, E. Psychotherapy and the patient with a limited life span. *Psychiatry*, 24:318-323, 1961.

LEVINE, M. A memo from ML. *Arch. Gen. Psychiat.*, 26:1-2, 1972.

LEVINSON, P. On sudden death. *Psychiatry*, 35:160-173, 1972.

LEVINSON, P. Obstacles in the treatment of dying patients. *Amer. J. Psychiat.*, 132:28-32, 1975.

LIEGNER, L. M. St. Christopher's Hospice, 1974. *JAMA*, 234:1047-1048, 1975.

LIFTON, R. J. The sense of immortality: On death and the continuity of life. *Amer. J. Psychoanal.*, 33:3-15, 1973.

LIFTON, R. J. *The Life of the Self. Toward a New Psychology*. New York: Simon & Schuster, 1976, p. 190.

LIPMAN, A. G. Drug therapy in terminally ill patients. *Amer. J. Hosp. Pharm.*, 32:270-276, 1975.

MADDISON, D. & RAPHAEL, B. The family of the dying patient. In: B. Schoenberg, A. C. Carr, D. Pereitz, and A. H. Kutscher (Eds.), *Psychosocial Aspects of Terminal Care*. New York: Columbia University Press, 1972, pp. 185-200.

MAHONEY, J. & KYLE, D. Personality characteristics of volunteers for thanatological research. *Omega*, 7:51-57, 1976.

MCINTOSH, J. Processes of communication, information seeking and control associated with cancer: A selective review of the literature. *Soc. Sci. and Med.*, 8:167-187, 1974.

MEYER, J. E. (1973) *Death and Neurosis*. New York: International Universities Press, 1975, p. 147.

MOUNT, B. The problem of caring for the dying in a general hospital; the palliative care unit as a possible solution. *Canad. Med. Assoc. J.*, 115:119-121, 1976.

MUSLIN, H. L., LEVINE, S. P., & LEVINE, H. Partners in dying. *Amer. J. Psychiat.*, 131:308-310, 1974.

NORTON, J. Treatment of a dying patient. *Psychoanal. Stud. Child*, 18:541-560, 1963.

PARKES, C. M. Evaluation of family care in terminal illness. Alexander Ming Fisher Lecture read at Columbia University, New York, 1975.

PATTISON, E. M. The experience of dying. *Amer. J. Psychother.*, 21:32-43, 1967.

PATTISON, E. M. Help in the dying process. In: S. Arieti (Ed.), *American Handbook of Psychiatry*, 2nd Edition, Vol. 1. New York: Basic Books, 1974a, pp. 685-702.

PATTISON, E. M. Psychosocial predictors of death prognosis. *Omega*, 5:145-160, 1974b.

PRESTON, C. E. Behavior modification. A therapeutic approach to aging and dying. *Postgraduate Med.*, 54:64-68, 1973.

QUINT, J. C. *The Nurse and the Dying Patient.* New York: Macmillan, 1967, p. 307.

RAMSEY, P. The indignity of "death with dignity." In: P. Steinfels and R. Veatch (Eds.), *Death Inside Out. The Hastings Center Report.* New York: Harper & Row, 1974, pp. 81-96.

RENNEKER, R. E. Countertransference reactions to cancer. *Psychosomat. Med.*, 19:409-418, 1957.

ROOSE, L. J. The dying patient. *Int. J. Psycho-Anal.*, 50:385-395, 1969a.

ROOSE, L. J. To die alone. *Ment. Hyg.*, 53:321-326, 1969b.

ROSENTHAL, H. R. Psychotherapy for the dying. *Amer. J. Psychother.*, 11: 626-633, 1957.

ROSENTHAL, H. R. The fear of death as an indispensable factor in psychotherapy. *Amer. J. Psychother.*, 17:619-630, 1963.

SAETHER, W. *Kvinnen, kroppen og angsten.* Oslo: Gyldendal, 1974, p. 170 (in Norwegian).

SANDFORD, B. An obsessional man's need to be "kept." *Int. J. Psycho-Anal.*, 33:144-152, 1952.

SANDFORD, B. Some notes on a dying patient. *Int. J. Psycho-Anal.*, 38:158-165, 1957.

SAUL, L. J. Reactions of a man to natural death. *Psychoanal. Quart.*, 28: 383-386, 1959.

SAUNDERS, C. Care of the dying. *Nursing Times Reprint.* London: Macmillan Company, 1959, p. 32.

SAUNDERS, C. *The Management of Terminal Illness.* London: Hospital Medicine Publ., 1967, p. 29.

SAUNDERS, C. A therapeutic community: St. Christopher's Hospice. In: B. Schoenberg, A. C. Carr, D. Peretz, and A. H. Kutscher (Eds.), *Psychosocial Aspects of Terminal Care.* New York: Columbia University Press, 1972, pp. 275-289.

SAUNDERS, C. Control of pain in terminal cancer. *Nursing Times*, 72:1133-1135, 1976a.

SAUNDERS, C. The nursing of patients dying of cancer. *Nursing Times*, 72: 1203-1205, 1976b.

SAUNDERS, C. M. (Ed.). *The Management of Terminal Disease* (The Management of Malignant Disease Series). London: Edward Arnold, 1978, p. 210.

SCHELL, H. W. Adrenal corticosteroid therapy in far-advanced cancer. *Geriatrics*, 27:131-141, 1972.

SCHULZ, R. & ADERMAN, D. Clinical research and the stages of dying. *Omega*, 5:137-143, 1974.

SEARLES, H. F. Schizophrenia and the inevitability of death. *Psychiat. Quart.*, 35:631-665, 1961.

SHELDON, A., RYSER, C. P., & KRANT, M. J. An integrated family orientated cancer care program: The report of a pilot project in the socioemotional management of chronic disease. *J. Chron. Dis.*, 22:743-755, 1970.

SHNEIDMAN, E. S. Orientations toward death: A vital aspect of the study of lives (Chap. 9). In: R. W. White (Ed.), *The Study of Lives*. New York: Atherton, 1963, pp. 201-227.

SHNEIDMAN, E. S. On the deromanticization of death. *Amer. J. Psychother.*, 25:4-17, 1971.

SHNEIDMAN, E. S. *Deaths of Man*. New York: Quadrangle/The New York Times Books, 1973, p. 238.

SHNEIDMAN, E. S. (Ed.). *Death: Current Perpectives*. Palo Alto, Ca.: Mayfield, 1976, p. 547.

SHNEIDMAN, E. S. Some aspects of psychotherapy with dying persons. In: Ch. A. Garfield (Ed.), *Psychosocial Care of the Dying Patient*. New York: McGraw-Hill, 1978, pp. 201-218.

SIMPSON, M. A. *Dying, Death, and Grief. A Critically Annotated Bibliography and Source Book of Thanatology and Terminal Care*. New York: Plenum Press, 1979, p. 288.

STEDEFORD, A. Psychotherapy of the dying patient. *Brit. J. Psychiat.*, 135: 7-14, 1979.

STERN, M. M. Fear of death and neurosis. *J. Amer. Psychoanal. Ass.*, 16: 3-31, 1968.

STOTLAND, E. *The Psychology of Hope: An Integration of Experimental, Social and Clinical Approaches*. San Francisco: Jossey-Bass, 1969, p. 234.

STRAUSS, A. L. & GLASER, B. G. *Anguish. A Case History of a Dying Trajectory*. Mill Valley, Calif.: The Sociology Press, 1970, p. 193.

STRAUSS, A. L., GLASER, B., & QUINT, J. The nonaccountability of terminal care. *Hospitals*, 38:73-87, 1964.

SUDNOW, D. *Passing On. The Social Organization of Dying*. Englewood Cliffs, N.J.: Prentice-Hall, 1967, p. 176.

TOYNBEE, A. and others. *Man's Concern with Death*. London: Hodder & Stoughton, 1968, p. 280.

TROMBLEY, L. E. A psychiatrist's response to a life-threatening illness. *Life-Threatening Behav.*, 2:26-34, 1972.

TRUAX, C. B. & CARKHUFF, R. R. *Toward Effective Counseling and Psychotherapy: Training and Practice*. Chicago: Aldine, 1967, p. 416.

TWYCROSS, R. G. The use of narcotic analgesics in terminal illness. *J. Med. Ethics*, 1:10-17, 1975.

TWYCROSS, R. G. Studies on the use of diamorphine in advanced malignant disease. Dissertation, University of Oxford, 1976, p. 117.

TWYCROSS, R. G. Relief of pain. In: C. M. Saunders (Ed.), *The Management of Terminal Disease*. London: Edward Arnold, 1978, pp. 65-92.

VACHON, M. L. S. Motivation and stress experienced by staff working with the terminally ill. *Death Education*, 2:113-122, 1978.

VACHON, M. L. S., LYALL, W. A. L., & FREEMAN, S. J. J. Measurement and management of stress in health professionals working with advanced cancer patients. *Death Education*, 1:365-375, 1978.

WAHL, C. W. The fear of death. *Bull. Menninger Clin.*, 22:214-223, 1958.

WAITZKIN, H. & STOECKLE, J. D. The communication of information about illness. Clinical, sociological and methodological considerations. *Adv. Psychosom. Med.*, 8:180-215, Basel: Kaker, 1972.

WALLACE, E. R. IV Thanatos—a reevaluation. *Psychiatry*, 39:386-393, 1976.

WEISMAN, A. D. *The Existential Core of Psychoanalysis: Reality Sense and Responsibility*. Boston: Little, Brown, 1965, p. 268.

WEISMAN, A. D. The patient with a fatal illness—to tell or not to tell. *JAMA*, 201:646-648, 1967.

WEISMAN, A. D. Misgivings and misconception in the psychiatric care of terminal patients. *Psychiatry*, 33:67-81, 1970.

WEISMAN, A. D. *On Dying and Denying: A Psychiatric Study of Terminality*. New York: Behavioral Publ., 1972, p. 247.

WEISMAN, A. D. *The Realization of Death. A Guide for the Psychological Autopsy*. New York: Jason Aronson, 1974, p. 207.

WEISMAN, A. D. Thanatology. In: A. M. Freedman, H. I. Kaplan, and B. J. Sadock (Eds.), *Comprehensive Textbook of Psychiatry*, 2nd Edition, Vol. 2. Baltimore: Williams & Wilkins, 1975, pp. 1748-1759.

WEISMAN, A. D. Early diagnosis of vulnerability in cancer patients. *Amer. J. Med. Sci.*, 271:187-196, 1976a.

WEISMAN, A. D. Coping behavior and suicide in cancer. In: J. W. Cullen, B. H. Fox, and R. N. Isom (Eds.), *Cancer: The Behavioral Dimensions*. New York: Raven Press, 1976b, pp. 331-341.

WEISMAN, A. D. The psychiatrist and the inexorable. In: H. Feifel (Ed.), *New Meanings of Death*. New York: McGraw-Hill, 1977, pp. 108-122.

WEISMAN, A. D. & HACKETT, T. P. Predilection to death: Death and dying as a psychiatric problem. *Psychosom. Med.*, 23:232-256, 1961.

WEISMAN, A. D. & HACKETT, T. P. Denial as a social act. In: S. Levin and R. J. Kahana (Eds.), *Psychodynamic Studies on Aging*. New York: International Universities Press, 1967, pp. 79-110.

WEISMAN, A. D. & KASTENBAUM, R. *The Psychological Autopsy. A Study of the Terminal Phase of Life*. New York: Behavioral Publ., 1968, p. 59.

WEISMAN, A. D. & WORDEN, J. W. Psychosocial analysis of cancer deaths. *Omega*, 6:61-75, 1975.

WHITMAN, H. H. & LUKES, S. J. Behavior modification for terminally ill patients. *Amer. J. Nursing*, 75:98-101, 1975.

WILMER, H. A. The doctor-patient relationship and the issues of pity, sympathy and empathy. *Br. J. Med. Psychol.*, 41:243-248, 1968.

WOLFF, K. Personality type and reaction toward aging and death. A clinical study. *Geriatrics*, 21:189-192, 1966.

WORBY, C. M. & BABINEAU, R. The family interview: Helping patient and family cope with metastatic disease. *Geriatrics*, 29:83-94, 1974.

WORDEN, J. W., JOHNSTON, L. C., & HARRISON, R. H. Survival quotient as a method for investigating psychosocial aspects of cancer survival. *Psycholog. Reports*, 35:719-726, 1974.

YOUNG, W. H. Death of a patient during psychotherapy. *Psychiatry*, 23:103-108, 1960.

ZINKER, J. C. & FINK, S. L. The possibility for psychological growth in a dying person. *J. Gen. Psychol.*, 74:185-199, 1966.

Name Index

273

Subject Index

**The
Institute
For
Psychoanalysis**

*180 N. MICHIGAN AVENUE
CHICAGO, ILLINOIS 60601*